"The concept of the glycemic index has been distorted and bastardised by popular writers and diet gurus. Here, at last, is a book that explains what we know about the glycemic index and its importance in designing a diet for optimum health. Carbohydrates are not all bad. Read the good news about pasta and even—believe it or not—sugar!"
—ANDREW WEIL, M.D., University of Arizona College of Medicine, author of
Spontaneous Healing and *8 Weeks to Optimum Health*

"Forget *Sugar Busters*. Forget *The Zone*. If you want the real scoop on how carbohydrates and sugar affect your body, read this book by the world's leading researchers on the subject. It's the authoritative, last word on choosing foods to control your blood sugar."
—JEAN CARPER, best-selling author of *Miracle Cures, Stop Aging Now!*
and *Food: Your Miracle Medicine*

"*The Glucose Revolution* is nutrition science for the 21st century. Clearly written, it gives the scientific rationale for why all carbohydrates are not created equal. It is a practical guide for both professionals and patients. The food suggestions and recipes are exciting and tasty."
—RICHARD N. PODELL, M.D., M.P.H., Clinical Professor,
Department of Family Medicine, UMDNJ-Robert Wood Johnson
Medical School, and co-author of *The G-Index Diet:
The Missing Link That Makes Permanent Weight Loss Possible*

"Here is at last a book explaining the importance of taking into consideration the glycemic index of foods for overall health, athletic performance, and in reducing the risk of heart disease and diabetes. The book clearly explains that there are different kinds of carbohydrates that work in different ways and why a universal recommendation to "increase the carbohydrate content of your diet" is plainly simple and scientifically inaccurate. Everyone should put the glycemic index approach into practice."
—ARTEMIS P. SIMOPOULOS, M.D., senior author of *The Omega Diet*
and *The Healing Diet* and President, The Center for Genetics,
Nutrition and Health, Washington, D.C.

Other Glucose Revolution Titles

The Glucose Revolution: The Authoritative Guide to the Glycemic Index—
The Groundbreaking Medical Discovery

■

The Glucose Revolution Pocket Guide to the Top 100 Low Glycemic Foods
The Glucose Revolution Pocket Guide to Diabetes
The Glucose Revolution Pocket Guide to Losing Weight
The Glucose Revolution Pocket Guide to Sports Nutrition
The Glucose Revolution Pocket Guide to Sugar and Energy
The Glucose Revolution Pocket Guide to Your Heart
The Glucose Revolution Pocket Guide to the Glycemic Index and Healthy Kids
The Glucose Revolution Pocket Guide to Children with Type 1 Diabetes

The
GLUCOSE
REVOLUTION
Life Plan

DISCOVER HOW TO MAKE THE GLYCEMIC INDEX—
THE MOST SIGNIFICANT DIETARY FINDING OF THE LAST 25 YEARS—
THE FOUNDATION FOR A LIFETIME OF HEALTHY EATING

Jennie Brand-Miller, Ph.D.

Kaye Foster-Powell, B.SC., M. Nutr. & Diet

Johanna Burani, M.S., R.D., C.D.E.

MARLOWE & COMPANY
NEW YORK

THE GLUCOSE REVOLUTION LIFE PLAN
Copyright © 2000, 2001 by Dr. Jennie Brand-Miller,
Kaye Foster-Powell and Johanna Burani

Recipes copyright © 2000 Lisa Lintner
Photographs on the 8-page color insert and on pages 7, 10, 51, 63, 70, and 129 are by Jennifer Soo;
   all other photographs copyright © Photodisc.

Published by
Marlowe & Company
An Imprint of Avalon Publishing Group Incorporated
841 Broadway, 4th Floor
New York, NY 10003

First published in Australia in 2000 under the title
The Glucose Revolution G.I. Plus
by Hodder Headline Australia Pty Limited.

This edition is published by arrangement
with Hodder Headline Pty Limited

Library of Congress Cataloging-in-Publication Data
    Brand-Miller, Janette, 1952-
        The glucose revolution life plan / by Jennie Brand-Miller,
    Kaye Foster-Powell, and Johanna Burani.
            p. cm.
        Includes Index.
        ISBN 1-56924-609-2
        1. Glycemic index. 2. Carbohydrates in human nutrition.
    I. Foster-Powell, Kaye. II. Burani, Johanna C. III. Title.

    QP701 .B73 2001
    613.2'83—dc21
                                            2001030025

9 8 7 6 5 4 3 2

Designed by Pauline Neuwirth, Neuwirth & Associates, Inc.

Printed in the United States of America
Distributed by Publishers Group West

CONTENTS

GET READY TO join the revolution: A revolution so profound and far-reaching that it will change the way you eat, the way you cook— even the way you think about food. We're talking about the glycemic index, a ranking of foods by their ability to raise blood sugar levels, which has become one of the most enduring and inspiring dietary concepts to arise in the last 20 years of the 20th century.

The fact is, the glycemic index, which started out as a dietary tool for people with diabetes, has come of age! It's the new way of eating that everyone's talking about—and one of the few programs around with years of scientific research to support it.

The dietary guidelines in this book are based wholly on *scientifically confirmed nutritional information*—expertise that's often scarce in other nutrition volumes. In *The Glucose Revolution Life Plan*, we explain the benefits of the glycemic index as they relate to the most up-to-date scientific findings—not on the anecdotal evidence from a few nutrition enthusiasts. What's more, *The Glucose Revolution Life Plan* gives you the whole package: It explains how the glycemic index fits in with other health messages about the different types of fat and protein and shows you how easy it is to expand your healthy eating choices.

If you've read *The Glucose Revolution* or any of the subsequent *Glucose Revolution Pocket Guides*, you already know that eating low G.I. foods can benefit everyone: You can control your diabetes, lower your risk of heart attack, keep your weight under control and improve your sports performance. In fact, the potential importance of the glycemic index in these areas is where research is now heading. And remarkably, many of the studies are now coming from here in the United States—one of the last bastions of opposition to the glycemic index.

Research has already shown that low G.I. foods:

- reduce the risk of heart disease, obesity and type 2 diabetes;
- help keep us from overeating;
- bring about lower **insulin**** levels, making our bodies burn fat more easily;
- help to lower blood fats;
- help people with diabetes to control their blood sugar levels; and
- may influence our heart disease risk as much as the type of fat we eat.

These facts are no exaggeration—they're confirmed by results of studies published in prestigious journals by scientists around the world.

But what if you've never read *The Glucose Revolution*? This book is for you, too! We'll give you all the information that you need to know: First, we'll review the basics so that you'll know how to use the glycemic index every day to eat healthier and feel better. We'll also show you how easy it is to expand these healthy eating choices.

Then, we'll take you beyond the basics by showing you the big picture. You'll discover how you can make the glycemic index—the most significant dictary finding of the last 25 years—the foundation for a lifetime of healthy eating, because we'll provide you with:

Note: All words in **boldface appear in the Glossary on pp. 230–233.

- details describing how *The Glucose Revolution Life Plan* can help you fight disease;
- easy-to-understand, scientifically validated information on the protein vs. carbohydrate debate;
- the real story behind dietary fat (hint: it's not *all* bad for you!);
- sample menus from Mediterranean countries and Asia so that you can enjoy a wide range of low G.I. foods' flavors and textures; and
- more than 60 great-tasting, easy-to-make, low G.I. recipes, including choices for appetizers, salads, entrees, snacks and desserts; and
- even more information about the glycemic index (including updated tables listing the glycemic index values of many popular foods).

You'll discover that this new, healthier way of eating is both easy and delicious!

**The glycemic index,
the most significant dietary finding
of the last 25 years, has come of age!**

Part One

THE GLUCOSE REVOLUTION PLUS

today's

nutritional needs

on one plate

CHAPTER 1

The Glucose Revolution

IF YOU'VE READ *The Glucose Revolution* and have been eating the low G.I way, you already know that you can reap tremendous health benefits from this new way of eating. If you aren't yet familiar with the glycemic index, or would like a quick refresher, we offer some highlights about what this revolutionary new way of eating can mean to you.

As we mentioned earlier, eating low G.I. foods can affect a wide range of diseases and conditions, including diabetes, heart disease and obesity. Below, we offer some frightening disease statistics and describe how using the glycemic index can help steer you clear of illness and tilt the good-health odds in your favor.

diabetes

Did you know that every day in the United States, more than 2,000 people are diagnosed with diabetes? And even more striking is the number of people who have the disease and don't even know it: In addition to the

10.3 million who have already been diagnosed with diabetes, another 5.4 million people remain undiagnosed—unaware that they're even sick! And in 1997, diabetes killed 62,636 Americans, and nearly 800,000 new cases of diabetes are diagnosed every year.

In fact, many people don't even know they are suffering from the seventh leading cause of death in the United States until they develop one of its life-threatening complications such as blindness, kidney disease, heart disease, stroke or nerve damage.

The Glucose Revolution Life Plan can help because:

■ We provide an easy and effective way to eat a healthy diet and control fluctuations in blood sugar.
■ We offer a lifestyle plan that includes many traditionally "taboo" foods (because they don't cause the unfavorable effects on blood sugar they were believed to have).
■ Diets containing low G.I. foods improve blood sugar control in people with both type 1 (insulin-dependent) and type 2 (non-insulin dependent) diabetes.

obesity

You can't go anywhere these days without people talking about what they're eating—and not eating. It seems everyone's uttering those five golden words: "I'm on a new diet." But would you believe that even with all those diets, the number of overweight and obese people in our society is actually climbing? In fact, one study found that 325,000 deaths in the U.S. each year can be attributed to obesity. That makes obesity the second leading cause of preventable death—surpassed only by smoking.

The problem is so pervasive that some studies find 55 percent of American adults weighing more than they should. Worse yet, if this trend continues, experts say that within just a few generations, every adult American will be overweight. And excess weight brings with it a host of other health problems, such as heart disease, diabetes, some types of cancer and high blood pressure.

If you're overweight (or consider yourself to be) chances are that you have looked at countless books, brochures, and magazines offering a solution to losing weight. At best, a weight-reducing "diet" will reduce your calorie intake. At worst, it will change your body composition for the fatter. The reason? Many diets teach you to reduce your carbohydrate intake to bring about quick weight loss. The weight you lose, however, is mostly water (that was trapped or held with stored carbohydrate) and eventually muscle (as it is broken down to produce glucose). Once you return to your former way of eating, you regain a little bit more fat. With each desperate repetition of a diet, you lose more muscle. Over a course of years, the resulting change in body composition to less muscle and more fat makes it increasingly difficult to lose weight.

By the way, within these pages, when we use the word *diet* we're talking about the foods you eat in general as well as specific foods that you should eat as part of a healthy lifestyle. We aren't referring to the popular use of the word *diet*: an attempt to lose weight by eating (or not eating) certain foods. *The Glucose Revolution Life Plan* can help because low G.I. foods:

- fill you up, keep you satisfied for longer, and help you burn more of your body fat and less of your body muscle;
- enable you to increase your food intake without increasing your waistline; and
- control your appetite.

heart disease

Heart disease is the single biggest killer of Americans. So big, in fact, that every 29 seconds an American will suffer either a heart attack or go into cardiac arrest. According to 1997 estimates, more than 59 million Americans have one or more forms of cardiovascular disease. What's more, in 1997, heart disease accounted for 41.2 percent of all deaths.

So what causes this deadly disease? It's often caused by **atherosclerosis** or "hardening of the arteries." Generally, people develop atherosclerosis gradually, and live much of their lives blissfully unaware of it. If the disease develops fairly slowly it may not cause any problems—even into great old age. But if its development is accelerated by one or more of many processes, the condition may cause trouble much earlier in life.

The Glucose Revolution Life Plan can help fight heart disease by:

- reducing blood cholesterol levels;
- increasing "good" **high-density lipoprotein (HDL) cholesterol;**
- helping you lose weight;
- reducing "bad" **low-density lipoprotein (LDL) cholesterol;** and
- increasing your body's sensitivity to insulin.

so . . . what is the glycemic index?

The glycemic index is a ranking of foods based on their immediate effect on blood sugar levels. Carbohydrate foods that break down quickly during digestion (we'll call them "gushers") have the highest G.I. values because their blood sugar response is fast and high. Carbohydrate foods that break down slowly, releasing glucose gradually into the bloodstream (we'll call these "tricklers"), have low G.I. values.

The substance that produces the greatest rise in blood sugar levels is pure glucose. The glycemic index of pure glucose is set at 100 and every other food is ranked on a scale from 0 to 100 according to its effect on blood sugar levels.

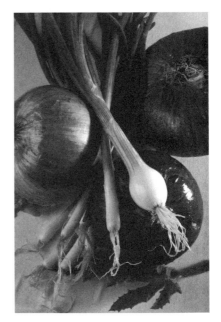

Today we know the G.I. values of hundreds of different foods that have been tested following the standardized method. The complete table of the G.I. values of hundreds of foods can be found in Part Four of this book, starting on page 216.

how the glycemic index came to be

The glycemic index concept was first developed in 1981 by a team of scientists led by Dr. David Jenkins, a professor of nutrition at the University of Toronto, Canada, to help determine which foods were best for people with diabetes. At that time, the diet for people with diabetes was based on a system of carbohydrate exchanges or portions, which was complicated and not very logical. The carbohydrate exchange system assumed that all starchy foods produce the same effect on blood sugar levels even though some earlier studies had already proven this was not correct. Jenkins was one of the first researchers to question this assumption and to investigate how real foods behave in the bodies of real people.

Jenkins's approach attracted a great deal of attention because it was so logical and systematic. When scientists, using Jenkins's technique, began to study the actual blood sugar responses to different foods in hundreds of people, they found that many starchy foods (such as some types of bread and potatoes) were digested into sugar and entered the bloodstream very quickly and that many sugar-containing foods, such as fruit and even some cookies, were not responsible for high blood sugars. That was quite a surprise!

Over the next fifteen years medical researchers and scientists around the world, including the authors of this book, tested the effect of many foods on blood sugar levels and developed a new concept of classifying carbohydrates based on their glycemic index.

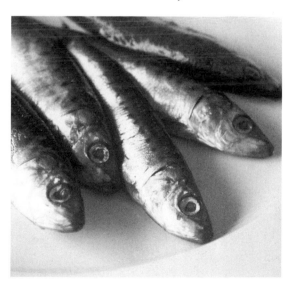

Key Factors That Influence the Glycemic Index

Cooking methods

Cooking and processing increases the glycemic index of a food because it increases the amount of gelatinized starch in the food. Here's what happens: When a food is exposed to water, the swelling (gelatinization) of starches increases, as does the food's surface area. That, in turn, increases the food's enzymatic activity, which increases the glycemic index.

Cornflakes, rice cakes and popcorn are all good examples of foods that have higher G.I. values when they're processed.

Physical form of the food

An intact fibrous coat on a food, such as that on whole grains and legumes, acts as a physical barrier (it takes longer for enzymes to break through the food's fibrous layers), slowing digestion and lowering a food's glycemic index.

Type of starch

There are two types of starch in foods, amylose and amylopectin. The more amylose starch a food contains, the lower the glycemic index. Examples of high-amylose foods include most legumes (kidney beans, chick peas and lentils) and several types of rice (Uncle Ben's converted, brown and basmati). Amylopectin, on the other hand, is a larger, more branched molecule. Its bonds are broken down more easily, causing faster digestion and giving the food a higher glycemic index.

Fiber

Viscous soluble fibers, such as those found in rolled oats and apples, slow down digestion and lower a food's glycemic index. (The more viscous a food is, the slower it moves through the gut, and the more slowly it gets digested.)

Sugar

The amount and type of sugar will influence a food's glycemic index. For example, fruits with a high concentration of naturally occurring fructose (such as apples and oranges) have a low glycemic index. Our bodies metabolize fructose in such a way that results in a slow release of glucose, lowering the glycemic index of a food.

sources of carbohydrate

Carbohydrate mainly comes from plant foods, such as cereal grains, fruits, vegetables and legumes (such as lentils and beans). Milk products also contain carbohydrate in the form of milk sugar or lactose, which is the first carbohydrate we eat as infants. Some foods contain a large amount of carbohydrate (cereals, potatoes, legumes and corn are good examples), while other foods, such as string beans, broccoli and salad greens, have very small amounts of carbohydrate. You can eat these foods freely, but they can't exclusively provide anywhere near enough carbohydrate for a high carbohydrate diet. And as nutritious as they can be, plain green salads aren't meals by themselves and should be complemented by a carbohydrate-dense food such as bread and a small portion of legumes or other low fat protein.

The following foods are high in carbohydrate and provide very little fat. Eat lots of them, but spare the butter, margarine and oil when you prepare them.

the best low fat, high carbohydrate choices

CEREAL GRAINS

These include rice, wheat, oats, barley, rye and anything made from them (bread, pasta, breakfast cereal and flour).

FRUITS

A few tasty examples are apples, oranges, bananas, grapes, peaches, and melons.

STARCHY VEGETABLES

Foods such as potatoes, corn, taro, and sweet potato help to create filling, satisfying meals.

LEGUMES, PEAS AND BEANS

Baked beans, lentils, kidney beans, and chickpeas are a few good low G.I. choices.

MILK

Not only is milk an excellent source of carbohydrate, it's also rich in bone-building calcium. (Adults should use low fat or skim milk and yogurt to minimize fat intake.)

high versus low G.I. foods

High G.I. foods (G.I. > 70; such as potatoes, Rice Krispies, processed breads) raise blood sugar levels the most.

Low G.I. foods (G.I. < 55; such as pasta, legumes, All Bran, old-fashioned oats) raise sugar levels least.

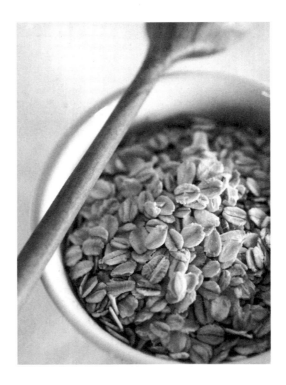

Substituting Low G.I. Foods For High G.I. Foods

We believe that the most appropriate and practical way to put the G.I. theory into practice is simply to substitute low G.I. foods for high G.I. foods, which lowers your diet's overall glycemic index.

As we mentioned above, some of the richest sources of carbohydrate include bread, crackers, cookies and baked goods, breakfast cereals, rice, pasta, potatoes and potato products. Choosing low G.I. varieties of these foods will significantly lower the glycemic index of your diet.

HIGH G.I. FOOD	LOW G.I. ALTERNATIVES
Bread	
Fluffy, light, smooth textured white or whole wheat (made from enriched wheat flour)	Dense breads containing a lot of whole grains; sourdough and stone ground flour breads (types that don't contain any enriched wheat flour)
Rice	
Short grain sticky (Chinese or Italian), jasmine	Long-grain basmati, imported Japanese, Uncle Ben's converted, brown, long-grain white
Potatoes	
Instant mashed, red- and white-skinned baking varieties	All pastas, noodles, legumes (including soybeans, kidney beans, lentils, chickpeas, baked beans), barley and bulgur (cracked wheat), sweet potato, yam, taro, new potatoes (these have a moderate glycemic index)

HIGH G.I. FOOD	LOW G.I. ALTERNATIVES
Cereals	
Most processed cold breakfast cereals, as well as quick and instant cooked types (such as oatmeal)	Rolled oats, semolina, muesli, granola, All Bran with Extra Fiber, Bran Buds, Grapenuts, Special K, oat bran
Crackers	
Most crackers (Saltines, Triscuits), rice cakes	Ryvita, stoneground wheat thins, WASA
Fruit	
Mango, pineapple, dates, watermelon, raisins	Apples, pears, citrus fruits, cherries, peaches, plums

The Impact of Insulin

The pancreas is a vital organ near the stomach, and its main job is to produce the hormone insulin. Carbohydrate stimulates the secretion of insulin more than any other component of food. The slow absorption of the carbohydrate in our food means that the pancreas doesn't have to work as hard, so it needs to produce less insulin.

If the pancreas is overstimulated over a long period of time, it may become "exhausted" and genetically susceptible people may develop type 2 diabetes. And even if you don't have diabetes, too-high insulin levels can be dangerous, because although our bodies need insulin for carbohydrate metabolism, too much of this hormone can have a profound effect on disease development: Medical experts now believe that high insulin levels are one of the key factors responsible for heart disease and hypertension. And since insulin also influences the way we metabolize foods, it helps determine whether we burn fat or carbohydrate to meet our energy needs, and ultimately determines whether we store fat in our bodies.

How Much Carbohydrate?

FOOD	PERCENTAGE OF CARBOHYDRATE PER 100 GRAMS
Apple	12
Baked beans	11
Banana	21
Barley	61
Bread	47
Cookie	62
Corn	16
Cornflakes	85
Flour	73
Grapes	15
Ice cream	22
Milk	5
Oats	61
Orange	8
Pasta	70
Peas	8
Pear	12
Plum	6
Potato	12–17
Raisins	75
Rice	79
Split peas	45
Sugar	100
Sweet potato	17
Water cracker	71

low G.I. eating

Low G.I. eating means emphasizing whole grains and legumes—barley, oats, dried peas and beans—in combination with certain types of breads, pasta, rice, vegetables and fruits. Stock your pantry with these foods and keep a loaf of low G.I. wholegrain bread in the freezer.

UNLIMITED VEGETABLES

You can eat most vegetables without thinking about their glycemic index. Most are so low in carbohydrate that they have no measurable effect on our blood sugar levels, but they still provide valuable amounts of fiber, vitamins and minerals. Higher carbohydrate vegetables include potato, sweet potato, corn and peas. Among these, corn and sweet potato are the lower G.I. choices.

Salad vegetables such as tomatoes, lettuce, cucumber, peppers and onions have so little carbohydrate that it's impossible to test their glycemic index values. In generous serving sizes, they will have no effect on blood sugars. Think of them as "free" foods that are full of healthful micronutrients. Eat and enjoy!

CEREALS AND GRAINS

Cereals and grains are the major source of energy and protein for many of us these days, but they weren't part of the diet that we evolved over millions of years. Archaeological findings of life 15,000 years ago herald the beginnings of our use of cereal grains for food. As populations increased, resources of mammals, fish and birds became depleted and the demand on agriculture increased. Over the past 10,000 years we have increasingly relied upon cereals for food. Our ancestors began processing cereals by grinding them between stones, which yielded small amounts of coarse meal. Later, we began to mill cereals using high-speed rolling machines, which yielded tons of fine white flour.

There are many nutritional implications of this change to our diets, one of which has been an increase in the glycemic index of the foods we eat. Modern cereal processing methods transform the low G.I. carbohydrate of cereal grains to high G.I. foods. In order to eat a low G.I. diet, we need to rely less heavily on processed cereal products and more on whole grain cereals.

BREADS

One of the most important changes you can make to lower your diet's glycemic index is to choose a low G.I. bread. Some good choices include:

WHOLE GRAIN BREADS

Whole grain breads contain lots of "grainy bits" and tend to be chewy. Where the fibrous seed coat of cereal grains is intact it acts as a physical barrier to slow starch digestion. In some wholegrain breads, the low glycemic index may also result from the long fermentation time during the dough's preparation. During this process the yeast consumes the quickly digested starch, converting it to energy, carbon dioxide (to make the bread rise) and a little alcohol, which evaporates during baking. What the yeast leaves behind is the more slowly digested starch.

PUMPERNICKEL

Pumpernickel is a true whole grain bread, because it's made from whole rye grains.

STONE GROUND FLOUR AND SPROUTED WHEAT

These have low G.I. values, probably because they contain coarsely milled and intact grains.

SOURDOUGH

In sourdough breads, lactic acid and propionic acid, produced by yeast's natural fermentation of starch and sugars, may lower a food's glycemic index by slowing stomach emptying.

CHAPATI (CHICKPEA FLOUR-BASED)

Chapati is an unleavened bread that's popular in India and on the Indian subcontinent. While it's often made with wheat flour, it's also made from chickpea flour (gram flour) or baisen, which is milled from a small variety of chickpeas. Chapati made from chickpea flour has a significantly lower glycemic index than that made from wheat flour because of the nature of the starch.

TORTILLAS (CORN-BASED)

These flat Mexican pancakes are made from ground dried corn kernels (cornmeal). You can also find tortillas made from wheat flour, but corn produces a lower glycemic index.

WHY ARE THERE NO G.I. VALUES FOR MEAT, NUTS AND AVOCADOS?

These foods contain either very little or no carbohydrate, so you can consider their glycemic index zero!

The Take Home Message

- Eating low G.I. foods is a good idea for everyone.
- Low G.I. foods result in slow and sustained release of sugar into the bloodstream.
- High G.I. foods result in quick release of sugar into the blood.

CHAPTER 2

Fats:
Facts and Fallacies

YOU CAN'T TURN on the television or open a newspaper these days without reading something about fat. The problem is, much of the information we're getting is either too scientific or too confusing. What's the bottom line? Is fat healthy or unhealthy?

The short answer: It depends. It's true that the type of fat you eat determines, to a large degree, whether you'll suffer a heart attack or stroke. What's more, the right type of fat in your diet (even if it's a low fat diet) may reduce your risk of certain types of cancer, depression, many autoimmune diseases such as arthritis, and may generally promote health and longevity. Indeed, there's good evidence that the type of fat an infant receives in its first few weeks of life may increase intelligence and learning ability!

One of the main findings of the past decade is that not all fats are bad for your heart; in fact, we all need to eat some fat for optimal health. In our quest for a non-fattening diet, though, we've unwittingly thrown out the baby with the bath water. Many of us decided that all fats were bad and that a healthy diet contained as little fat as possible. Not true! In reality, it's possible to replace the harmful fats with the beneficial ones, which allows you to consume as much as 35 to 40 percent of your calories as fat. For many people, higher fat diets taste better, and they're easier to stick with, since a diet higher in heart-healthy fats more closely matches our early eating habits, ingrained since childhood.

some facts about fats

Fatty acids are described as **saturated, monounsaturated or polyunsaturated**, which is determined by their molecular structure. The most important thing to remember about dietary fats is this: Saturated fats are heart-unhealthy, while unsaturated fats (mono- and polyunsaturated) are heart-healthy.

Fats In A Nutshell

All fats and oils contain differing amounts of the following:
- Monounsaturated fats, or MUFAs;
- Polyunsaturated fats, or PUFAs; and
- Saturated fat.

MUFAS	PUFAS	SATURATED FATS
Heart healthy	Heart healthy	Heart un-healthy
Lower LDL	Lower LDL	Increase LDL
Protect HDL	Lower HDL	
Food sources:	**Food sources:**	**Food sources:**
Olive oil, canola oil, avocados, peanut butter, almonds, pistachios	Salmon, sardines, mackerel, bluefish, canola oil, walnuts, flaxseed, white albacore tuna	Full-fat dairy products, fatty cuts of meat, poultry skin

---

Concealed Fats In The Foods We Eat

Many people these days are reducing their fat intake by using less fat in food preparation, choosing low fat dairy foods and buying leaner cuts of meat. But is this the best we can do? Although these are healthy habits, much of the fat we eat is coming from foods that we don't prepare ourselves. Here are a few examples:

FOOD	FAT (GRAMS)
Wise potato chips, lunch pack:	10
Small chocolate milkshake (10 ozs.):	11
Small chocolate bar (1.5 ozs.):	14
Ben & Jerry's peanut butter ice cream (1/2 cup):	25
Cheese danish:	22
2 plain doughnuts:	22
Movie-type popcorn (large container):	24
Quaker 100% Natural Oats and Honey Granola (1 cup):	18
Container of ramen noodle soup:	14
Big Mac and large fries:	54
Taco Bell's Supreme Chicken Fajita and Bell Grande Nachos:	64
Sweet and sour pork with fried rice:	35 (minimum)
Fettuccine alfredo (2 cups) and garlic bread slice (2 ozs.):	54
KFC's Chunky Chicken Pie:	42

The message? If you don't know how much fat a food contains, it's best to eat very little of it, or avoid it altogether.

the "good" fats

As we mentioned earlier, you may be surprised to learn that some fats are good for you. For example, **monounsaturated fats**, or **MUFAs**, such as those in olive and canola oils, can reduce the risk of cardiovascular disease by reducing **triglycerides** in the blood and increasing levels of good HDL cholesterol. (This is especially important if you have diabetes or a family history of heart disease.) Research has shown that a low HDL level is one of the best predictors of increased risk of heart attack.

The best types of fat to consume are those that contain a high proportion of monounsaturated (MUFAs), **polyunsaturated (PUFAs)** and **omega-3 fatty acids**. In practice, this means you should prepare meals with lean meat, seafood, olive oil, canola oil and peanut oil, because they all contain a lot of monounsaturated fatty acids. You can also include nuts, avocados and polyunsaturated oils such as safflower oil and sunflower oil. These foods and oils should take the place of saturated fats, such as you find in fatty meat, fried foods, high fat dairy products and most bakery products. Many of the recipes in Part Three of this book can help you achieve the ideal fatty acid proportions in your diet.

Polyunsaturated fats (PUFAs) include omega-3 and omega-6 fatty acids; both are essential in your diet. Research suggests that we should be eating more omega-3s than omega-6s, but we're not—in fact, though we need both types of fatty acids in our diet, many experts believe that we're eating too much of the omega-6s. We'll describe these two omega fats in greater detail in Chapter 3.

Polyunsaturated margarines and seed oils, such as safflower, sunflower and soybean oils, are the major sources of omega-6 fatty acids in most of our diets. Fish and other seafood are the main source of omega-3 fatty acids, as is canola oil.

The table on pages 35 and 36 shows the amounts of saturated fatty acids, and omega-6 and omega-3 fatty acids in various fats and oils.

ESSENTIAL FATTY ACIDS

Not only are some types of fat good for you, but also your body actually requires some types of fats—called **essential fatty acids**—which you can only get through your diet. We used to think a very small amount of these fatty acids would suffice, but we were wrong: We appear to need much larger amounts of them because they play a fundamental role in the development of our cell membranes, and we also need them to grow and develop normally.

The human brain requires two of the most important essential fatty acids, **eicosapentanoic acid (EPA)** and **docosahexanoic acid (DHA).** Both of these essential fatty acids are omega-3s, which we'll discuss in more detail in Chapter 3. Without EPA and DHA our body tissues can suffer, causing a high tissue turnover rate. The earliest sign of this high turnover rate would be scaly dermatitis (skin irritation), and we die if the deficiency exists for longer than a few months. But that's not all: We also appear to need essential fatty acids to achieve the best of mental health and to reach our full intellectual potential. Science has proven that depression is linked to a lack of these special fatty acids in our diet.

The best sources of EPA and DHA are seafood, especially "fatty" fish, such as salmon, mackerel, sardines and herring (which, in truth, are actually no fattier than lean meat, but do contain more fat than most other fish). Our absolute dependency on these fatty acids may go all the way back to our evolutionary ancestors, who ate large amounts of fish and shellfish.

═══ *Dairy Foods: A Mixed Blessing* ═══

Though dairy foods are a rich, readily absorbed source of calcium, they can be high in saturated fat. To meet calcium requirements, experts recommend that adults eat two to three servings of dairy products every day. Good low fat dairy choices include skim or 1 percent milk and nonfat or low fat yogurts.

If you're lactose intolerant, try calcium-fortified orange and grapefruit juices, lactose reduced milk, high-calcium soy milk, salmon (canned, with bones), high-calcium tofu, calcium-fortified breakfast cereal and dried figs — all great-tasting nondairy sources of calcium.

Many experts believe that infants don't get enough EPA and DHA in infant formulas and therefore recommend supplements. Breast milk is a good source of these special fatty acids, and Japanese women, whose normal diet includes lots of fish, produce milk with the highest essential fatty acid levels of all.

The "Bad" Fats

Most people have heard that **saturated fat** isn't good for us, and there's no argument from anybody on this point. Solid at room temperature, saturated fat comes in the form of fatty marbling in meat, the cream in milk and other high fat dairy products, and in some of the tropical oils such as palm oil, widely used as shortening for frying and for making cakes, pies, cookies and crackers. Many studies from all around the world have clearly shown that saturated fat increases our risk of coronary heart disease. But don't make the mistake of thinking animal foods are all bad just because some contain saturated fat. In fact, as we explain in Chapter 6, humans evolved on a steady diet of animal foods and we are dependent on them to get many of the nutrients we need. In our evolutionary past, however, animal foods were not as high a source of saturated fat as they are now. Game meat, even today, is lower in fat and has relatively less saturated fat compared with that of domesticated animals.

When animals are confined so that they can't move around naturally and are over-fed a diet of grains, they gain excess body fat in and around the muscles. Grain-fed meat is typically what we find in America today: It's highly marbled (that is, it has fat within the muscle tissue that's impossible to avoid eating) and, to most Americans, this means high quality, good-tasting meat. Though it may taste good, it's extremely high in saturated fat, and may increase your risk of heart disease, obesity and certain cancers. Fats from other animals (including pigs and chickens) are less saturated and contain some polyunsaturated fatty acids. Fats from deer and other game animals are lower still in saturated fats and often contain significant amounts of polyunsaturated fatty acids.

Recently, researchers have found that **trans-fatty acids** are just as bad for our health as saturated fats. Trans-fatty acids are produced during the manufacture of margarines and behave like saturated fat in the products (increasing its firmness), as well as in our bodies (increasing the risk of heart attack). Foods high in trans fats include fried fast foods, some margarines, crackers, cookies and snack cakes.

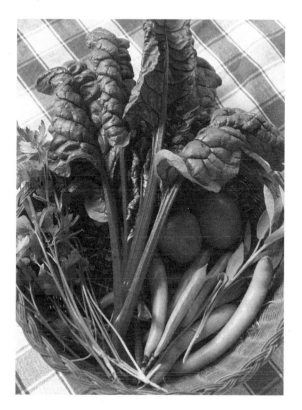

═══ *Is Vegetable Oil A Friendly Fat?* ═══

We used to think—thanks to many of the television commercials in the 1960s and '70s—that all vegetable oils are good for us. While it's true that all vegetable oils are cholesterol free, their fatty acids can be highly saturated, promoting high blood cholesterol. Coconut and palm oils, for example, are highly saturated vegetable fats. Most other plant oils, on the other hand, contain little saturated fat; for example, avocado, peanut and other nut oils are largely monounsaturated, making them heart-healthy.

For The Love Of Cheese

Having a hard time finding a tasty low fat cheese? Try these tips for making the most of your higher-fat cheese choices.

- Consider eating a little of a strong-flavored cheese rather than a lot of something bland and tasteless.

- Shave some fresh Parmesan on your pasta. It's delicious and super high in calcium.

- Enjoy full fat cheeses in small amounts. This includes regular types of cheddar, American, Swiss, brie, Colby, cream cheese, gouda and havarti.

- Try grating hard cheeses to make them go further.

- Serve your favorite soft cheeses with low fat crackers, and fresh and dried fruit.

- Try some mozzarella cheese—whole milk or part skim—it may contain less fat than some reduced-fat cheeses. Use it in recipes and sandwiches.

- Feel free to use lower fat cheeses, such as cottage cheese, ricotta and feta daily.

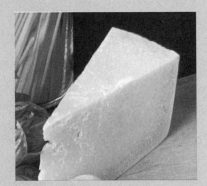

our recommended intakes

Health experts advise us to increase our carbohydrate intake to about 55 percent of our total calories and to choose low G.I. versions of the high carbohydrate foods. The remaining calories in our diet (45 percent of it) should be split between protein and fat. Chances are that you're eating at least 15 percent of your energy as protein—most people eat this amount without even trying. This still leaves plenty of room for some fat: In fact, most experts consider a diet "low fat" if no more than 30 percent of total calories come from fat. It's not necessary to eat less fat than this, especially when you consume heart-healthy monounsaturated fats (MUFAs), which have important health effects. It's important not to throw out the healthy fats with the unhealthy ones—and that's exactly what many people have been doing in their quest for the ultimate low fat diet.

which oil for what?

Try using a variety of different oils, depending on the dish:

- For stir fries, add a distinctive flavor with canola-based flavored oils or peanut or sesame oil. You can also drizzle a little sesame oil over the top of the stir fry for added flavor.
- For salad dressings you can add a nutty flavor with walnut or macadamia oil, or use some sesame oil for an oriental salad.
- For Mediterranean cooking, including salads, use extra virgin olive oil for its distinctive flavor.
- For everyday cooking, including roasting and frying, choose a neutral-flavored oil with a high smoke point, such as sunflower or canola. Looking for a pleasant nutty flavor in baked goods? Try corn oil.

Fats And Food Label Claims

So convincingly are foods marketed these days that many of us automatically reach out for that package or bottle that carries the word "light." Supermarket shelves contain light oil, margarine, butter, jam, cheese, chocolate, crackers, cookies, cakes—the list goes on and on. But it pays to be informed about what food-label claims actually mean.

Prior to the regulations mandated by the Food and Drug Administration's (FDA's) 1990 Nutrition Labeling and Education Act, food manufacturers could decide the portion sizes they used for the "Nutrition Facts" on their food labels. To make a product appear lower in calories or fat or sodium, for example, the serving sizes they used were often unrealistically small. Now the FDA has leveled the playing field by regulating standardized serving sizes that all food manufacturers need to use. Here's what the words really mean:

▶ Low fat:

The food must not contain more than 3 grams of fat per serving. For example, low fat or 1 percent milk contains about 2.5 grams of fat per 8 ounce serving.

▶ Reduced fat/less fat/fewer:

Foods with any of these words on the label contain 25 percent less of a nutrient than the regular product. For example, reduced-fat Swiss cheese contains 25 percent less fat than regular cheese. (Keep in mind, though, that this doesn't necessarily make it a low fat food.)

▶ Fat free:

These foods contain less than 0.5 grams of fat per serving.

▶ Cholesterol free:

To be labeled "cholesterol free" a food must not contain more than 2 milligrams of cholesterol and 2 grams of saturated fat. Canola oil, like most vegetable oils, is an example.

Fats And Food Label Claims

▶ **Light or lite:**

These words may only refer to the color or flavor of a food (although by law this should be clear from the label). It may also refer to fewer calories (33 percent fewer), or less fat (50 percent less) or less sodium (50 percent less). Be careful when choosing reduced-fat "light" foods: They may have about the same number of calories as their regular counterparts, thanks to additional carbohydrate.

▶ **Lean:**

Meats with "lean" on the label contain less than 10 grams of fat, 4 grams of saturated fat, and 95 milligrams (mg) of cholesterol per serving.

▶ **Extra lean:**

These meats have less than 5 grams of fat, 2 grams of saturated fat and 95 mg of cholesterol per serving.

═══ *The Take Home Message* ═══

- A "low fat diet" does not mean a "no fat diet."
- It is better to avoid saturated fat than to avoid all fats.
- Choose lean meat and low fat dairy products.
- Be aware of concealed fats in foods.

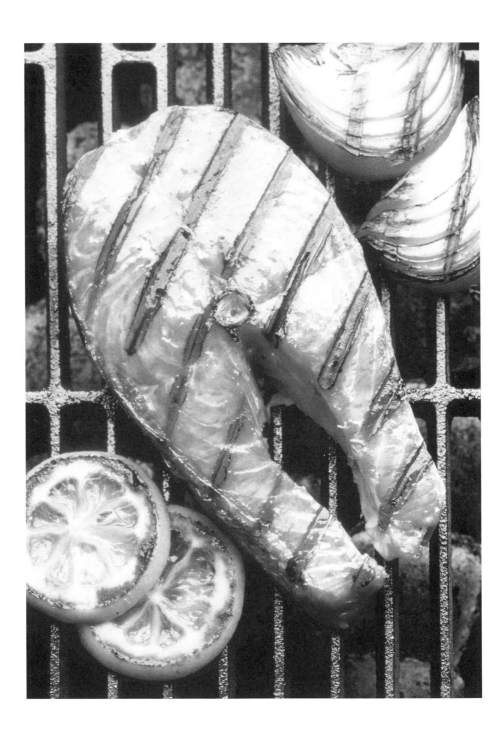

CHAPTER 3

The Omega Story

OMEGA-3 FATS, one of the most important good-for-you fats, are polyunsaturated fatty acids found in several plants and plant oils, including canola, peanut, flaxseed and soy. They're found in even greater quantities in fatty fish and seafood. Since foods containing these fats are so beneficial to health, we've included many of them in the Glucose Revolution Life Plan recipes in Part Three.

Several studies have shown that if you eat fish regularly you could reduce your risk of coronary heart disease. In fact, studies have found that eating just one serving of fish a week could reduce your risk of a fatal heart attack by 40 percent! (Eating fish more often than once a week doesn't seem to increase this protective effect.) The likely protective components of fish are the long-chain marine omega-3 polyunsaturated fatty acids called eicosapentanoic acid (EPA) and docosahexanoic acid (DHA), the essential fatty acids that we mentioned in Chapter 2. The omega-3 fatty acid derived from plants, **alpha-linolenic acid** or **ALA** (one source of which is canola oil), may also decrease the risk of heart attack, but the effect is not as strong as with the fatty acids from fish. Many experts believe that many of our diets are relatively deficient in omega-3 fatty acids.

how omega-3s help

Omega-3 fatty acids are essential for normal growth and development, and may play an important role in the prevention and treatment of heart disease, hypertension, arthritis and cancer. Scientists are still trying to work out how omega-3 fatty acids help to prevent heart attacks. To be sure, consuming more omega-3 fats reduces several risk factors, for example:

- At high doses, marine omega-3 fatty acids have been shown to lower triglyceride levels in the blood, and high triglyceride levels are a recognized risk factor for heart disease.
- Omega-3s may also slightly raise levels of HDL—the good cholesterol—in the blood. (These effects are specific to marine sources of omega-3 fats; experts don't see the same effects with the plant omega-3 fatty acids.)
- Some studies suggest that marine omega-3 fatty acids reduce blood clotting. Although we want blood to clot quickly when we're bleeding, if it tends to coagulate excessively, clots could form inside our blood vessels, a condition called thrombosis. One of the common precipitating events of a heart attack is when blood clots form in the heart's arteries, which can completely cut the blood supply to a vital part of the heart muscle. The heart then loses its ability to pump blood to the brain, causing death. Clots in less important arteries can mean that you survive the attack but the risk of having another is high.
- Omega-3 fats may also reduce your susceptibility to an irregular heartbeat, known as heart arrhythmia or ventricular fibrillation, which is one of the main causes of sudden death after an acute heart attack. Studies have shown that omega-3 fatty acids help to restore regular beating in isolated heart cells.
- High intakes of omega-3 fatty acids can also reduce high blood pressure (also called hypertension). However, scientists only find this effect when people consume large amounts of fish oil supplements, not the quantities that you might consume just from eating fish.

Omega-3 Fats And Your Health

Arthritis relief

In clinical trials, marine omega-3 fatty acids consistently reduce the pain and morning stiffness that's associated with rheumatoid arthritis. Certain substances in the blood, called **eicosanoids** and **cytokines**, initiate the immune response and its consequent inflammation. Scientists believe that omega-3 fatty acids decrease these reactions.

Brain development

Omega-3 fatty acids help nerve growth in fetuses and young infants. Some experts believe that infants are not able to synthesize enough docosahexanoic acid (DHA) for optimal growth from the precursor compound alpha-linolenic acid (ALA). Breast milk, however, is naturally rich in DHA, and DHA levels in the brains of breast-fed babies are higher than those in formula fed babies.

Formulas enriched with DHA have been found to improve visual acuity and neuromental development in premature infants compared with conventional formula, but the long-term implications of adding DHA to formula are unknown, so some infant formula manufacturers are unwilling to risk the safety of the formula by adding it. This is yet another reason why we should feed all babies human milk whenever possible.

Pregnant and lactating women can increase their intake of omega-3s by eating more fish; they will pass the benefit on to their infants either through the placenta or in their breast milk.

Cancer risk

Many studies show an association between high fish consumption and reduced risk of colon and breast cancer. In addition, animal experiments have shown that high doses of fish oils inhibit the development of chemically-induced mammary (breast) and colorectal cancers. Experts say, however, that the current evidence is insufficient to prove that eating fish decreases cancer risk.

does the ratio of omega-3 to omega-6 fatty acids matter?

Experts disagree about the importance of the ratio of omega-3 to omega-6 fats in our diets. Some believe the ratio is too low: that we eat too few omega-3s and too many omega-6s from safflower and sunflower oils and their margarines. Many researchers agree that the ratio of omega-6s to omega-3s should be 1:4 or 1:1 at the most. That is, you should consume about four times more omega-3s than omega-6s, but certainly no more omega-6s than omega-3s.

concerns with omega-3 fats

One of the concerns scientists have with omega-3 fatty acids is that they oxidize, or turn rancid. Oxidized fats have been implicated in causing arteriosclerosis, or hardening of the arteries. In fact, all polyunsaturated fats (PUFAs) are susceptible to oxidation, so we should consume them with adequate amounts of **antioxidants** such as vitamin E. Fortunately, both PUFAs and vitamin E tend to occur together in the same foods, including: polyunsaturated plant oils such as margarines, salad dressings, green and leafy vegetables, wheat germ, whole grain products, liver, egg yolks, nuts and seeds.

In their natural state, all PUFAs are rich sources of vitamin E, but sometimes food processing can inadvertently reduce antioxidant (such as vitamin E) concentrations, which is one reason why we should avoid foods and oils that have been stored for long periods of time—even in the freezer—or under inappropriately high temperatures. Oils are usually packaged in dark containers to protect against light, which increases chances of rancidity.

Omega Fats In A Nutshell

Omega-6 (Linoleic Acid)

Our bodies can't make linoleic acid, so we must get it from the foods we eat. We need this fatty acid for cell membrane integrity, blood pressure regulation, blood clot formation, regulation of blood **lipids** and immune response to injury and infection.

Good food sources: Leafy vegetables, seeds, nuts, grains, vegetable oils (corn, safflower, soybean, cottonseed, sesame, sunflower)

Omega-3 (Linolenic Acid)

Like linoleic acid, linolenic acid is also essential to our bodies, is not produced by our bodies and, therefore must come from food. Omega-3s aid in brain development, bring arthritis pain relief and may lower cancer risk.

Good food sources: Fats and oils (canola, soybean, walnut, wheat germ, some margarines), nuts and seeds (butternuts, walnuts, soybean kernels), soybeans

EPA (Eicosapentanoic Acid) and DHA (Docosahexanoic Acid)

Since our bodies only make small amounts of **EPA** and **DHA**, we must rely on getting these fatty acids from our diets, especially from fish and seafood. EPA helps nerve growth in fetuses and young infants and DHA has been found to improve visual acuity and neuromental development in premature infants.

Good food sources: Human milk, shellfish, mackerel, tuna, salmon, bluefish, mullet, sturgeon, anchovy, herring, trout, sardines

the conclusion

There's more than enough evidence to suggest that marine omega-3 fatty acids can be good for your health—especially for people with coronary heart disease. Plant and marine sources of omega-3s have distinct physiological effects, so they cannot replace each other. Try to eat fish at least once a week, and include a plant source of omega-3s, such as canola oil, in your diet. (Olive oil is not a rich source of omega-3 fatty acids.) To increase the plant omega-3 fatty acids further, aim to eat green leafy vegetables every day.

═══ *The Best Fish Sources Of Omega-3 Fats* ═══

Both canned and fresh fish are rich sources of omega-3 fats. The following lists show some of the richest varieties:

CANNED FISH
Salmon (including pink and red)
Sardines
Mackerel
White albacore tuna

FRESH FISH
Atlantic and Pacific salmon (fresh or smoked)
Mackerel (Atlantic, Pacific, Spanish)
Sea mullet
Southern bluefin tuna
Swordfish

SHELLFISH
Eastern and Pacific oysters
Squid (calamari)

POLYUNSATURATED FAT CONTENT OF FOODS

The health benefits of omega-3 and omega-6 polyunsaturated fatty acids (PUFAs) are widely acknowledged. The table below lists the total omega-6 and omega-3 fatty acid content of foods, and gives an estimate of the amount of omega-3 PUFAs that will be derived from the alpha-linolenic acid content (omega-3 equivalent) of these foods.

Abbreviations

tr = trace   wt = weight   av = average

TYPE OF FOOD	OMEGA-6 FATTY ACIDS (G)	OMEGA-3 FATTY ACIDS (G)	LONG CHAIN OMEGA-3 FATTY ACID EQUIVALENT (G)
Fats, spreads and oils			
Beef dripping, 1 tbsp	0.4	0.2	0.02
Blended polyunsaturated oil, 1 tbsp	8.6	1.2	0.2
Butter, regular, 1 tbsp	0.3	0.1	0.02
Butter, reduced-fat, 1 tbsp	0.1	0.05	0.01
Canola oil, 1 tbsp	3.6	1.8	0.3
Corn oil, 1 tbsp	9.4	0.4	0.05
Cottonseed oil, 1 tbsp	10.4	0.0	0.0
Flaxseed (linseed) oil, 1 tbsp	2.9	10.3	1.5
Ghee (clarified butter), 1 tbsp	0.3	0.2	0.03
Lard, 1 tbsp	1.5	0.02	0.003
Corn oil, 1 tbsp	9.7	0.1	0.02
Margarine, polyunsaturated, regular, 1 tbsp	6.3	0.2	0.04
Margarine, polyunsaturated, reduced-fat, 1 tbsp	3.1	0.1	0.02
Olive oil, 1 tbsp	1.8	tr	tr
Palm oil, 1 tbsp	1.8	tr	tr
Peanut oil, 1 tbsp	6.1	0.4	0.05
Safflower oil, 1 tbsp	13.9	0.0	0.0

POLYUNSATURATED FAT CONTENT OF FOODS

TYPE OF FOOD	OMEGA-6 FATTY ACIDS (G)	OMEGA-3 FATTY ACIDS (G)	LONG CHAIN OMEGA-3 FATTY ACID EQUIVALENT (G)
Soybean oil, 1 tbsp	9.7	1.4	0.2
Sunflower oil, 1 tbsp	11.9	tr	tr
Sunola oil, 1 tbsp	1.4	0.0	0.0
Tallow, 1 tbsp	0.9	0.0	0.0
Salad dressings			
Coleslaw dressing, 1 tbsp	3.7	0.02	0.003
Coleslaw dressing, reduced-fat, 1 tbsp	1.2	0.02	0.003
French dressing, 1 tbsp	2.8	0.1	0.02
Italian dressing, 1 tbsp	3.8	0.02	0.003
Mayonnaise, 1 tbsp	5.7	0.03	0.005
Mayonnaise, reduced-fat	3.7	0.03	0.005
Thousand Island dressing, 1 tbsp	2.8	tr	tr
Eggs			
Egg, whole, raw, 1 egg	0.4	0.05	0.05
Egg, yolk, chicken, 1 yolk	0.6	0.07	0.05
Milk & dairy products			
Brie, 1 small wedge	0.1	0.06	0.01
Buttermilk, cultured, 1 cup	0.0	0.0	0.0
Cheddar cheese, 1-oz. cube	0.16	0.12	0.02
Cottage cheese, 1 tbsp	0.04	0.02	0.003
Cottage cheese, low fat, 1 tbsp	0.0	0.0	0.0
Cream, pure, 1 tbsp	0.2	0.06	0.01
Cream cheese, 1 tbsp	0.1	0.06	0.01
Edam cheese, 1-oz. cube	0.12	0.10	0.02

POLYUNSATURATED FAT CONTENT OF FOODS

TYPE OF FOOD	OMEGA-6 FATTY ACIDS (G)	OMEGA-3 FATTY ACIDS (G)	LONG CHAIN OMEGA-3 FATTY ACID EQUIVALENT (G)
Feta cheese, 1-oz. cube	0.12	0.10	0.02
Ricotta cheese, 1 tbsp	0.04	0.02	0.003
Swiss cheese, 1-oz. slice	0.18	0.10	0.02
Goat's milk, 1 cup	0.3	0.0	0.0
Ice-cream, premium, 1 tbsp	0.06	0.03	0.005
Ice-cream, natural, vanilla, ½ cup	0.20	0.12	0.02
Milk, low fat (0.2% fat), 1 cup	0.0	0.0	0.0
Milk, reduced-fat (1.4% fat), 1 cup	0.0	0.0	0.0
Milk, skim (0.1 % fat), 1 cup	0.0	0.0	0.0
Milk, full-cream (3.8% fat), 1 cup	0.3	0.0	0.0
Soy milk, (3.5% fat), 1 cup	5.4	0.0	0.0
Soy beverage, unfortified, 1 cup	2.8	0.3	0.04
Sour cream, regular, 1 tbsp	0.1	0.06	0.01
Sour cream, light, 1 tbsp	0.06	0.04	0.01
Yogurt, fruit, full-fat, 8 ozs.	0.2	0.0	0.0
Yogurt, fruit, low fat, 8 ozs.	0.0	0.0	0.0
Yogurt, plain, full-fat, 8 ozs.	0.2	0.0	0.0
Yogurt, plain, reduced-fat, 8 ozs.	0.0	0.0	0.0
Meats			
Beef, lean, 1 steak, 5 ozs.	0.2	0.09	0.06
Chicken breast, no skin, 3 ozs.	0.1	0.03	0.03
Lamb leg, 3 ozs.	0.1	0.08	0.05
Sausage, pork, 3 ozs.	1.3	0.1	0.1
Turkey, no skin, 1 slice, 2 ozs.	0.2	0.02	0.02
Turkey, with skin, 1 slice, 2 ozs	.0.5	0.04	0.02
Turkey loaf, 1 slice, 3 ozs.	0.7	0.05	0.02

POLYUNSATURATED FAT CONTENT OF FOODS

TYPE OF FOOD	OMEGA-6 FATTY ACIDS (G)	OMEGA-3 FATTY ACIDS (G)	LONG CHAIN OMEGA-3 FATTY ACID EQUIVALENT (G)
Fresh and canned fish			
Anchovy, canned in oil, drained,	50.3	0.2	0.1
Cod, 1 medium fillet, 4 ozs.	0.1	0.4	0.4
Crabmeat, canned in water, drained, 5 ozs.	0.06	0.1	0.1
Flounder, 4 ozs.	0.1	0.3	0.2
Lobster, cooked, 1 cup	0.1	0.3	0.3
Mackerel, fresh, 5 ozs.	0.2	1.2	1.1
Mackerel, canned, 1 cup	0.4	4.9	4.0
Mullet, 3 ozs.	0.2	0.7	0.6
Octopus, 4 ozs.	0.03	0.7	0.7
Orange roughy, 5 ozs.	0.3	0.4	0.4
Oyster, 12 raw	0.1	0.8	0.6
Perch, 4 ozs	0.2	0.5	0.4
Porgy, 1 fillet, 5 ozs.	0.1	0.6	0.6
Prawns, 5 cooked	0.05	0.1	0.1
Salmon, Atlantic, 5 ozs.	0.9	3.2	2.8
Salmon, pink, canned, 1 cup	0.2	3.1	2.8
Salmon, red, canned, 1 cup	0.3	3.7	3.2
Sardine, canned, 5 sardines	1.6	2.4	2.1
Scallop, 1 cup cooked	0.03	0.2	0.2
Shark, 5 ozs.	0.1	0.4	0.4
Skate (Ray), 5 ozs.	0.1	0.5	0.5
Snapper, 4 ozs.	0.1	0.4	0.4
Squid, 1 cup	0.03	0.4	0.4
Trout, rainbow, 4 ozs.	0.4	0.7	0.6
Tuna, southern bluefin, with skin, 5 ozs	.0.3	1.7	1.6

POLYUNSATURATED FAT CONTENT OF FOODS

TYPE OF FOOD	OMEGA-6 FATTY ACIDS (G)	OMEGA-3 FATTY ACIDS (G)	LONG CHAIN OMEGA-3 FATTY ACID EQUIVALENT (G)
Tuna, canned in oil, 1 cup	0.1	1.3	1.2
Whiting, 1 fillet, 2 ozs.	0.1	0.2	0.2
Nuts and seeds			
Almonds, 1/2 cup	10.8	0.0	0.0
Brazil nuts, 1/2 cup	2.5	0.0	0.0
Cashews, 1/2 cup	5.7	0.0	0.0
Coconut, dried, 1 cup	0.5	0.0	0.0
Coconut, fresh, 3 large pieces	0.2	0.0	0.0
Hazelnuts, 1/2 cup	4.9	0.1	0.01
Macadamia nuts, 1/2 cup	0.7	0.0	0.0
Nuts, mixed, salted, 1/2 cup	11.3	0.0	0.0
Peanuts with skin, 1/2 cup	12.2	0.0	0.0
Peanut butter, 1 tbsp	4.1	0.0	0.0
Pecans, 1/2 cup	13.3	0.3	0.05
Pine nuts, 1 tbsp	5.6	0.0	0.0
Pistachios, 1/2 cup	10.0	0.0	0.0
Sesame seeds, 1 tbsp	3.2	0.0	0.0
Sunflower seeds, 1 tbsp	5.5	0.0	0.0
Tahini paste, 1 tbsp	5.6	0.02	0.003
Walnuts, 1/2 cup, chopped	23.8	3.5	0.5

The figures in this table have been adapted from data for 100-gram portions listed in the following reference: Meyer, B. J., Tsivis, E., Howe, P. R. C., Tapsell, L. & Calvert, G. D., "Polyunsaturated Fatty Acid Content of Foods: Differentiating Between Long and Short Chain Omega-3 Fatty Acids," *Food Australia*, vol. 51, pp. 81-95, 1999.

The Take Home Message

- Try to include more omega-3 fats in your diet to reduce your risk of heart disease.
- Choose canola oil for cooking and salad dressings because of its high omega-3 content.
- Eat fish once a week, especially those varieties containing high levels of omega-3s, such as salmon and tuna.

CHAPTER 4

The Benefits of Mediterranean-style Diets

IN A WORLD where some people still don't get enough to eat, we in industrialized nations tend to suffer the effects of over-nutrition—too much food for our sedentary lifestyles and too many foods that have been linked to cardiovascular disease or excess weight. Because fat is the most calorically dense nutrient—yet can be less satisfying than either carbohydrate or protein—most experts think that high fat diets cause weight gain and its resulting diseases, including high blood pressure and diabetes. That's why American dietary guidelines emphasize the importance of eating a low fat diet. In fact, many people view fat—no matter what type—as the dietary villain. We now know, though, that this view oversimplifies the issue and that a healthy, balanced diet must contain some fat. But the *type* of fat you eat is extremely important.

In the 1980s, scientists were surprised to learn that the rates of heart disease and cancer in parts of Greece, where the traditional diet consisted primarily of fish, fruits, vegetables, olives and olive oil, were low compared to heart disease and cancer rates in North America, Europe and other parts of the world. Research since then has shown that a

Mediterranean-style diet can lower cholesterol and blood pressure and, therefore, the risk of heart disease. Experts think the **Mediterranean diet** is healthy not only because it's lower in saturated fat and higher in monounsaturated fats, but also because it's rich in **micronutrients** (such as folate, which we'll mention later) that reduce the risk of heart disease.

Not coincidentally, this Mediterranean eating style fits seamlessly into the Glucose Revolution Life Plan, because the low G.I. way of eating includes lots of fruits, veggies, grains, nuts, fish and some lean meat.

the seven countries study

A series of important studies, collectively called the Seven Countries Study, found that countries with low saturated fat intake, such as Japan and rural Mediterranean areas in southern Europe, had much lower rates of coronary disease than countries where saturated fat intake was higher, such as in the United States and northern Europe. There was no relationship, though, between total fat intake and coronary disease; that is, high total fat intake did not increase disease risk. Why? Because Mediterranean diets are low in dangerous saturated fat and high in heart-healthy monounsaturated fatty acids (MUFAs), which accounted for the high total fat intake. In addition, Mediterranean diets are full of fiber-rich fruits and vegetables and potentially protective nutrients called **phytochemicals**.

═══ *Monounsaturated Fatty Acids (MUFAS)* ═══

Monounsaturated fats can reduce the risk of cardiovascular disease by reducing blood triglycerides and increasing levels of good HDL cholesterol.

You can get more MUFAs by eating pistachios, peanut butter, canola oil, olives, olive oil, cashews, pecans, almonds and avocados.

It's interesting to note that the lowest rate of coronary disease was in Crete, which has the highest intake of total fat—nearly all of it from olive oil. Japan also has very low heart disease rates, which coincide with a low total fat intake. So both Japan and Crete could be considered two models of healthy eating: one (Japan's) based on rice, soy and fish and *low* in fat, the other (Crete's) based on cereals, vegetables, fish and olive oil and *high* in fat. We'll look at both models in this and the following chapter.

A 25-year follow-up of the Seven Countries participants continued to show very low heart disease rates in Japan and rural areas of southern Europe. Rates of colon, prostate and breast cancer, all high in northern Europe, the United States and Australia, are low in both Crete and Japan.

mediterranean-style diets and fat intake

One reason people who eat typical Mediterranean diets have low heart disease rates is likely because their diet has a positive impact on cholesterol levels. Many studies have shown that reducing saturated fat intake and replacing it with either carbohydrates or unsaturated oils lowers blood concentrations of bad LDL cholesterol—a firmly established cause of hardening of the arteries. Replacing saturated fats with carbohydrate, however, can negatively affect heart health by lowering good HDL cholesterol, the good cholesterol that helps to keep LDL cholesterol from accumulating in artery walls. (Lower HDL concentrations are associated with higher heart disease rates.) MUFAs, on the other hand, *don't* lower HDL cholesterol.

the micronutrient connection

Some of the micronutrients in Mediterranean-style diets may reduce disease rates, too. One of these micronutrients is folate, which is found in organ meats and green leafy vegetables. This vitamin is in short supply in many diets, and too little of this nutrient results in high levels of an amino acid called **homocysteine** in the blood. (Although we don't know

$\mathcal{M}ost$ $pasta$ is made from semolina (finely cracked wheat), which is milled from very hard wheat with a high protein content. A stiff dough, made by mixing the semolina with water, is forced through a die and dried. There is very little disruption of the starch granule during this process and the strong protein-starch interactions inhibit starch gelatinization. The dense consistency also makes the pasta resistant to disruption in the small intestine and contributes to the final low glycemic index—even pasta made from fine flour (instead of semolina) has a relatively low glycemic index. There's some evidence that thicker pasta has a lower glycemic index than thin types because of its dense consistency and perhaps because it cooks more slowly. (It's also less likely to be overcooked.) The addition of egg to fresh pasta lowers the G.I. value by increasing the protein content: Higher protein levels slow stomach emptying, because only about 60 percent of the protein gets broken down; the rest goes into storage as fat.

Italians eat their pasta "al dente" which literally means "to the tooth." It must be slightly firm and offer some resistance when you're chewing it. Not only does al dente pasta taste better than soft, soggy pasta, but it also has a lower G.I. value, because overcooking pasta increases starch gelatinization (or swelling) and boosts its glycemic index.

why or how, high levels of homocysteine are associated with a high risk of heart disease.) Folate-rich diets lower blood levels of homocysteine.

Diets high in fruit and vegetables also provide antioxidants that protect blood lipids and other compounds from oxidation. As we mentioned earlier, oxidized cholesterol is more likely to lead to hardened arteries.

the dash diet

High blood pressure (also called hypertension) is another risk factor for heart attack and stroke. Research shows that people who eat lots of vegetables tend to have lower blood pressure and suffer fewer strokes. In fact, the **Dietary Approaches to Stop Hypertension (DASH)** study found that very high fruit, vegetable and nut intakes reduced blood pressure. And the results in mildly hypertensive patients were astounding, far exceeding the results of other non-drug treatments (such as low-salt diets) and similar to results from drug therapy. Italian studies have also found that Mediterranean-style diets lower blood pressure.

should you eat a low fat or mediterranean diet?

There is a widening divide in the nutrition and public health community between those people who advocate a low fat diet and those who promote a higher-fat Mediterranean-style diet. As a result, most people receive conflicting and confusing information. Our view is that the optimal diet can be either low fat (as in Japan, which we'll talk about in the next chapter) or Mediterranean-style (as in Crete). In either case, you should be eating less saturated fat and fewer high G.I. carbohydrates. We leave the diet you choose strictly up to you—both are well suited to the Glucose Revolution Life Plan. Judging from the very low incidence of heart disease and cancer in the Mediterranean and parts of Asia, both traditional diets have the potential to dramatically benefit all of us!

It can be argued that one of the reasons for the success of a Mediterranean style diet is because it doesn't contain many high glycemic index foods, so glucose and insulin responses are reduced. In fact, in some studies, high carbohydrate-low G.I diets (which included foods such as pasta and legumes) had positive effects on blood lipids.

dietary recommendations for diabetes: high or low carbohydrate?

There is concern among some scientists that high carbohydrate diets are especially harmful for people with diabetes, so some experts recommend a high fat, high MUFA diet instead. Is this advice justified? The aim of diabetes management is to normalize blood sugar and lipid levels to prevent the short- and long-term complications of diabetes, particularly heart disease. (People with diabetes are three to four times more likely to die of a heart attack than people without the disease, even when cholesterol levels and blood pressure are the same.) To help lower heart disease risk, experts have long advised people with diabetes to reduce their saturated fat intake. If you lower your intake of saturated fat, however, you need to replace those calories with some other nutrient. So . . . protein, MUFAs, carbohydrate or PUFAs: Which should it be?

high protein diets

For most people with healthy kidneys, there may be some advantages to a higher protein intake, which we'll describe in Chapter 6. If you have diabetes, though, experts don't recommend that you eat a very high protein diet because it could hasten kidney problems, such as chronic renal failure. Most people with diabetes are at increased risk of developing kidney disease anyway, because high blood sugars put stress on the kidney's filtering mechanisms: The kidney's job is to filter waste products as it saves nutrients from the blood. It retains the sugars in the blood as best it can, but if blood sugars are highly concentrated, the kidneys can't keep up and those excess sugars are lost into the urine. (The presence of sugar in the urine is often how diabetes is first diagnosed.) If kidney function has deteriorated because of the excess sugar in the urine, the added stress of filtering the waste products of a high protein diet could be the straw that breaks the camel's back. For this reason, some experts recommend low-protein diets for people with diabetes who have renal complications.

high mufa diets and glucose control

As we mentioned earlier, experts debate about how we should replace our saturated fat calories. Should we switch to more carbohydrates or to

MUFAs? If you have diabetes, the current nutritional recommendations suggest that you can interchange carbohydrate and MUFAs, with the proportions determined by individual needs and desires. Some experts argue in favor of allowing a higher MUFA intake because they say that high carbohydrate diets can increase blood glucose and insulin concentrations, which result in high triglycerides and low HDL levels in the blood—changes that cause arteries to harden and increase the risk of coronary heart disease.

But it is best to wholeheartedly recommend a diet based on high MUFAs for people with diabetes? First, the American Diabetes Association doesn't consider the source of the carbohydrate (that is, a food's glycemic index) when discussing high carbohydrate diets. Many dietary trials have shown that lowering the glycemic index of dietary carbohydrate (with no change in total amount) improves blood glucose control by an average of 10 percent—the same amount of change we see when we treat type 2 diabetes with either oral medications or insulin.

Second, though high MUFA diets lower blood sugar and insulin responses after meals (because each meal contains less carbohydrate), there is no evidence that they improve *overall* blood sugar control, because fat is not broken down into glucose. In other words, a high MUFA meal results in lower glucose *after that meal*. But if other meals (with or without snacks) produce higher glucose levels, MUFAs may not impact the overall glucose average, or glucose control. By contrast, high carbohydrate-low G.I. diets lower blood sugar consistently.

Third, we see the positive effects of high MUFA diets on blood fats only when the high MUFA diet is extremely high in fat—as much as 45 to 50 percent of total calories—and very low in carbohydrate (about 35 percent of calories). In studies with smaller and more realistic dietary changes, the effects of MUFAs on blood lipids are quite modest. What's more, very high fat diets may promote insulin resistance and weight gain. (For more on this subject, see "High Fat Diets May Promote Weight Gain" on page 48.)

Furthermore, the effects of MUFAs on triglycerides have been shown in people with normal triglycerides, not in diabetes patients with high triglycerides. It is not logical to extrapolate from one to the other.

MUFAs may be useful, though, in the treatment of high blood lipids in people with diabetes—as long as they're also eating a low fat diet. In fact, scientists have found that diets containing 30 percent total calories from fat with a high proportion of MUFAs produce modest improvements in HDL and triglycerides.

mufas and weight control

Several studies suggest that diets high in MUFAs (high in olive and canola oil and nuts, for example) are just as effective as high carbohydrate diets when it comes to weight loss. In these studies, however, researchers strictly controlled the number of calories people were consuming as they added more MUFAs. The trouble is, if you start adding more MUFAs to your diet without regard to the number of calories you're taking in, you're likely to gain weight. And since weight loss is a primary treatment goal for most people with type 2 diabetes, and because America is currently in the midst of an obesity epidemic, some experts are cautious about recommending high MUFA diets without asking people to also control their daily calorie intake.

high fat diets may promote weight gain

It seems commonsensical that high fat diets can make you gain weight, and there are several theories to explain how it could happen. Experts believe that our bodies are capable of using carbohydrates, protein and fat as fuel. To maintain a steady weight, we must burn the same amount of calories from each of these nutrients (protein, fat and carbohydrate) as we consume. Unfortunately, at least as far as weight control is concerned, we have a much greater capacity to store ingested fat than we do either protein or carbohydrate. So our bodies prefer to store dietary fat and to burn carbohydrate and protein. Every day we burn virtually all of the carbohydrate and most of the protein calories that we've eaten.

Ingested calories from fat, on the other hand, will remain within our body's fat stores, unless, at a time when we need calories but eat no food, they're released into the blood as free fatty acids. (Given the statistics of the growing obesity problem in America, this situation apparently doesn't happen very often.) The sad reality is that the more fat we consume, the more our fat stores will expand to accommodate it—and with an almost limitless capacity to do so.

The combination of high fat and high G.I. carbohydrate may be a particularly fattening combination, because the high insulin response induced by high G.I. carbohydrates tells our bodies to burn more carbohydrate and less fat: In fact, one of insulin's most powerful actions is to switch off the release of free fatty acids from the fat stores. So as long as insulin levels are raised, our bodies will store (and keep storing) dietary fat rather than burn it.

The same scenario applies even if you have type 1 diabetes and don't produce insulin: Our bodies don't care where the insulin comes from, as long as it's there to do the job. If you have type 1 diabetes and your blood glucose numbers are high, you'll need more and more insulin to bring your numbers down. Here's what happens: If you have consistently high glucose numbers, your body can become more insulin resistant over time, making it require more "outside" insulin to produce the same glucose numbers that your body used to achieve with less insulin. Although this process doesn't happen overnight, it does happen frequently.

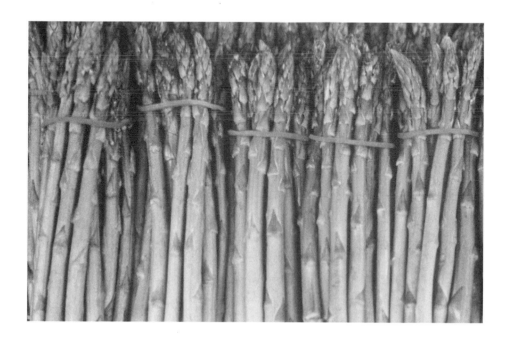

insulin resistance

Many of us have chronically high insulin levels because we're insulin resistant: that is, our bodies resist the normal actions of insulin. To overcome this insulin resistance, our bodies produce more and more insulin to move the glucose out of the bloodstream and into the muscles, where it is burned. Over the course of the day, our insulin levels increase, so we end up burning more carbohydrate and less fat, which some experts believe encourages increasing fat storage over time.

Compounding the problem, the carbohydrate stores in our bodies are thought to act as hunger barometers: When stores are low we feel hungry (whether or not we have burned the calories that we've previously eaten); when they're high, we feel satisfied. But if carbohydrate stores fluctuate widely throughout the day under insulin's influence, the net effect may be an excess intake of calories, causing us to gain weight.

fats won't fill you up

Another explanation for why high fat diets can encourage us to gain weight is because fats are less satiating (filling) than we once thought. Scientists have studied the "staying power" of ingested fat calories: After a high fat meal or snack, people consistently ate a significant number of calories, sometimes after only an hour!

As a result of studies such as these, scientists now say it's very easy for many of us to unintentionally consume too much fat. This could be one of the most important findings in nutrition science over the past decade, because it has turned upside down the general belief that fat is particularly filling. As we've just pointed out, the opposite is true. Of course a high fat meal can make you feel full, even sickeningly so. The trouble is, you already will have eaten an excessively large number of calories before your brain registers how full you are. After all, we all know how easy it is to quickly demolish a bag of potato chips or peanuts!

a word about low fat foods

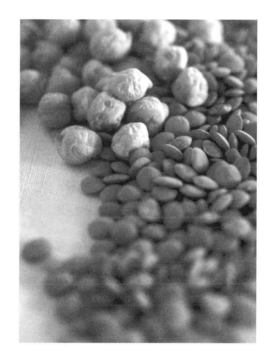

It's generally true that high fat foods contain more calories than low fat, high carbohydrate foods; for example, one ounce of peanuts contains 170 calories (and 69 percent fat), while an ounce of jellybeans contains only 100 calories and no fat. But this isn't always true—and it's becoming increasingly common to find low fat or fat-free foods on the market that have as many calories as their full-fat counterparts.

In fact, some low fat flavored foods contain even more calories than the full-fat versions. For example, one Kellogg's low fat strawberry Pop Tart contains 192 calories, while Pillsbury's regular strawberry breakfast pastry contains 180 calories. Why? Because the low fat food contains extra carbohydrate to create a creamy texture. The added carbohydrate compensates for the reduced amount of fat, both in texture and number of calories.

In addition, experts suggest that many of us interpret the words "low fat" on a food label as a license to eat more, and as a result, we may consume twice as many calories. This calorie overload may partly explain why more of us are becoming obese in the United States, despite the fact that we're eating less fat.

other health concerns

Increasing your intake of MUFAs to more than 35 percent of total calories may improve your triglyceride and HDL levels, but is inconsistent with dietary guidelines for the public, and with dietary guidelines to prevent cancer and heart disease. Remember that modifying the source of carbohydrate (by using low G.I. foods) could have the same beneficial effect as increasing MUFA intake, without the potential problems of increased fat intake.

the mediterranean diet

The Mediterranean diet contains lots of low G.I. carbohydrates—pasta, beans and fruit in particular—and people often eat meals with a salad and vinaigrette, which also lowers the glycemic index of a meal. You can reduce white bread's potentially high glycemic index if you eat it with low G.I. foods.

As long as total fat intake isn't too high (that is, no more than 30 to 35 percent of total calories), everyone—including people with diabetes—is likely to benefit from a Mediterranean-style diet. Compare the G.I. values of common carbohydrate foods in American diets with those of Mediterranean diets (below).

WESTERN DIET	G.I. VALUE	MEDITERRANEAN DIET	G.I. VALUE
WHITE BREAD	70	WHITE BREAD	70
POTATO	80-100	PASTA	40
BREAKFAST CEREAL	70-80	LEGUMES	20-30
COOKIES	60-70	FRUIT	30-40

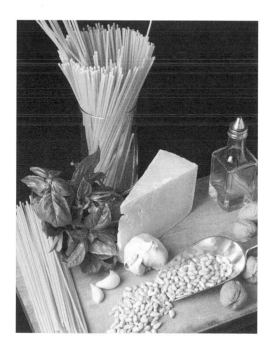

the glucose revolution life plan
mediterranean style menu

ADAPTING OUR DIET TO THE MEDITERRANEAN WAY OF EATING

The Mediterranean diet contains an abundance of plant foods including vegetables, fruits and legumes. Olive oil is part of the daily diet, and people eat fish more frequently than red meat. Because alcoholic beverages are a traditional part of meals in the Mediterranean, a glass of red wine has been included with the main meal.

You'll notice that these menus downplay the emphasis on eating low fat in favor of including more monounsaturated fats. Most of the carbohydrate has a low glycemic index.

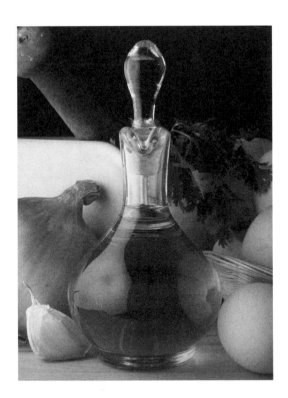

Note: For the menus below, follow the portion sizes listed in "What is a Serving?" on page 83.

the glucose revolution life plan mediterranean-style menu

Breakfast
Italian semolina toast with reduced-fat feta or mozzarella cheese
Large piece of seasonal fruit
Latte (made with espresso coffee and nonfat milk)

Lunch
Pasta (cooked al dente) with pesto sauce and sundried tomatoes
Large green bean, cucumber and tomato salad with vinaigrette dressing
Fresh fruit salad
Sparkling water

Dinner
Couscous pilaf
Broiled lemon sole
Steamed asparagus with sherry vinegar sauce
Small apple compote with chopped walnuts
One glass of red wine

The Take Home Message

- You can benefit from a Mediterranean-style diet, even if you have diabetes, as long as you aren't overweight.
- Remember that Mediterranean-style diets consist of more than just a lot of olive oil.
- If you have diabetes, avoid a high protein-low fat diet until we know more about its effects on renal function.
- Choose legumes, pasta, salad vegetables and vinegar dressings as an integral part of your Mediterranean-style diet.

CHAPTER 5

The Benefits of Asian-style Diets

PEOPLE LIVING THROUGHOUT Asia have low rates of heart disease, type 2 diabetes and cancer, and are less likely than people in some Western countries to become overweight or obese as they age. Why? It could be because they eat healthy, high fiber, high carbohydrate diets and get lots of physical activity. **Asian-style diets** contain a good deal of rice; in fact, people in Asian countries consume rice—usually white—in large amounts at all meals. (This eating style fits in perfectly with the Glucose Revolution Life Plan, since along with the rice, people in much of Asia also eat small amounts of some lean meat, poultry or fish, as well as vegetables and fruits.) In India, one low fat, low G.I. food, mashed legumes or dhals, often accompanies meals. Many **Asian-style diets** are low in fat (Indian food is one exception), and relatively rich in omega-3 fats. Japanese people, for example, regularly eat fish and seaweed, both good sources of omega-3 fats.

There are other benefits to Asian-style diets, too. Because meat and fish are so expensive, Asian people usually include lots of soybeans, other vegetables and sometimes seaweed with their rice. From a health perspective, these additional vegetables may be the most important component of the Asian diet, since vegetables are full of micronutrients such as antioxidants, vitamins, minerals and phytochemicals such as **isoflavones** and **phytoestrogens**.

Another plus: Traditional Asian recipes, which include lots of vegetables, fiber and tofu, make eating heart-healthy cancer-preventive meals easy and tasty!

the benefits of high fruit and vegetable intake

Five million years ago, the ancestors of the first hominids lived in the rainforests of Africa. Their diet was based on fruits, nuts, berries and insects and supplemented with animal food. Although the tables turned and animal food began to dominate as humans evolved, we have inherited the need for large amounts of the substances found in fruit and vegetables to promote good health. In fact, there's overwhelming evidence that fruits and vegetables play an important role in disease—especially cancer—prevention. The evidence is stronger for vegetable consumption and for raw, rather than cooked, foods.

Scientists have been researching the protective factors in fruits and vegetables for many years. Here are some of the key players:

- **Carotenoids.** Among the most well known phytochemicals, carotenoids are found in yellow and orange fruits and vegetables, as well as in dark green leafy vegetables. They are heart-healthy and may help to prevent certain cancers.
- **Lycopene.** This chemical gives tomatoes and pink grapefruit their red pigment, and has strong anti-cancer and antioxidant properties.
- **Indoles.** Found in cruciferous vegetables such as broccoli, cauliflower, cabbage and Brussels sprouts, indoles may reduce breast cancer risk.
- **Flavonoids and genistein.** Especially prevalent in soy foods, these phytochemicals help to prevent tumor formation.

- **Vitamin C.** This antioxidant vitamin abounds in many types of produce including strawberries, oranges, grapefruit, broccoli and green peppers.
- **Vitamin E.** This antioxidant vitamin plays a role in heart health; good food sources include vegetable oils, nuts and seeds.
- **Selenium.** A mineral often grouped with antioxidants, selenium may be cancer protective.

These protective factors may work by:

- binding with and diluting cancer-causing substances in the gut;
- offering antioxidant effects;
- stimulating detoxifying enzymes;
- inhibiting the formation of **nitrosamines**; and
- altering the metabolism of hormones.

It's more than likely that it is the combined effect of these substances that is responsible, rather than any one component. So don't be tempted to take a multivitamin supplement to replace a high intake of fruit and vegetables—you won't find all of the protective substances in a pill.

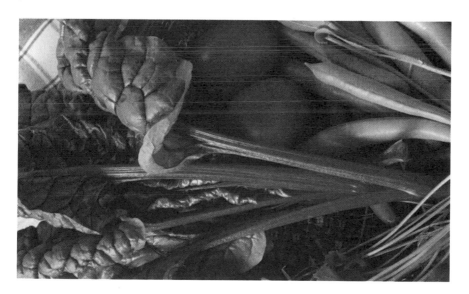

avoiding cancer

Can your diet prevent cancer? No one can answer that question better than the panel of the American Institute for Cancer Research (AICR) scientists who issued a landmark report on diet and cancer in 1997, called "Food, Nutrition and the Prevention of Cancer: A Global Perspective." The researchers of this nonprofit organization analyzed more than 4,500 studies conducted worldwide and estimated that if people would eat five or more servings of fruits and vegetables every day, overall cancer rates could drop by at least 20 percent!

New cancer cases are turning up far too rapidly around the world, and our country is no exception. Cancer is America's second leading cause of death, causing approximately 600,000 deaths a year. With such high stakes, the AICR scientists urge all Americans to take just a few simple steps to lower their cancer risk (see box above). Their recommendations summarize the best ways to prevent cancer—potentially for half a million people each year—in the United States alone.

the benefits of soy

Scientists believe that soybeans, and products made from them, such as tofu, protect Japanese, Chinese and other Asian populations from developing the high rates of heart disease and breast cancer that normally plague Western populations. In many Asian countries, people eat soy—a staple food—in many forms, including soy milk, soy sauce, soy flour, tofu and tempeh. Research suggests that soy foods help to reduce high blood lipid levels.

Some studies suggest that the isoflavones in soybeans are responsible for reducing the risk of breast cancer; they're thought to counteract the action of estrogen in pre-menopausal women. Some women, especially those who are overweight, are thought to produce too much estrogen, which stimulates the growth of abnormal breast tissue. Soy products are one of the best dietary sources of these isoflavones—or phytoestrogens, as they are often called.

Soybeans have one of the lowest G.I. values of any food. When you add them to meals and snacks, you reduce the overall glycemic index of your diet and gain important health benefits.

SOYBEANS

AVERAGE G.I. VALUE: 18

Soybeans and soy products have been a staple part of Asian diets for thousands of years and are an excellent source of protein. They're also rich in fiber, iron, zinc and vitamin B. They are lower in carbohydrate and higher in fat than other legumes but the majority of the fat is polyunsaturated. Just a quarter cup of soybeans can contribute a beneficial amount of the plant form of omega-3 fat.

Soy is also a rich source of phytochemicals, phytoestrogens in particular, which are plant estrogens with a structure similar to the female hormone estrogen, but with a much weaker action. The specific phytoestrogens in soy are known as isoflavones: The two main types are genistein and **daidzein**.

Many studies associate these isoflavones with improvements in blood cholesterol levels, relief from menopausal symptoms and lower rates of cancer.

Here are a few ways to incorporate more soy into your diet:

- Use canned soybeans in place of other beans in any recipe.
- Drink soy milk—it comes in plain, vanilla, chocolate and cappuccino flavors.
- Use "okara"—the drained soybean pulp that's the by-product of soy milk—as a thickener in baking.
- Cut firm tofu into cubes, marinate them in soy sauce, ginger and garlic, and add them to stir-fries. Or thread them onto kebabs for a barbecue.
- Include soybean oil or light, low-sodium soy sauce in your stir fries.
- Use silken tofu as a base for cheesecakes, creamy sauces and salad dressings.
- Substitute soy flour for half a cup of wheat flour in baked goods.
- Use roasted soy nuts in granola and salads or eat them as a snack in place of peanuts. (Look for unsalted or lightly salted products.)

which type of rice should you eat?

Because rice is the predominant carbohydrate source in Asia, its glycemic index determines to a large degree the overall glycemic index of the Asian-style diet. Rice varies markedly in its glycemic index, depending on the variety and the amount of starch it contains. Those varieties with more amylose have lower G.I. values: Amylose is a straight-chain starch molecule that tends to line up with itself in rows, forming tight bonds that make it less likely to gelatinize (expand with water) during cooking. Compared with amylopectin, a branched-chain starch, amylose starch needs higher temperatures and longer cooking times to gelatinize. Because the starch isn't fully gelatinized during cooking, higher amylose rice has a lower glycemic index.

Some rices, such as glutinous or sticky rice, contain only amylopectin with no amylose at all. As a result, the texture of the rice is quite different—the individual grains of rice stick to each other, hence the name "sticky" rice. On the other hand, rices with a high amylose content retain more of their individual integrity: It's possible to pick up the individual grains.

ADAPTING OUR DIET
TO THE ASIAN WAY OF EATING

Asian-style diets differ from Western diets in many ways, one of which is the proportion of plant to animal foods. In this menu, the protein content comes more from plants than from animal sources, and the rice and noodles keep the carbohydrate content high.

Note: For the menus below, follow the portion sizes listed in "What is a Serving?" on page 83.

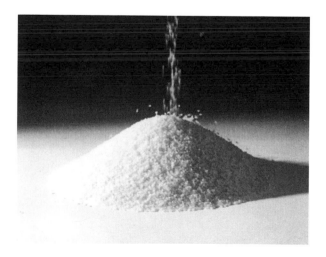

THE G.I. VALUES OF RICE

PRODUCT	G.I.	COMMENT
Basmati rice	58	Long grain rice with an aromatic flavor that develops with storage. Its higher amylose content (35 per cent of the starch is amylose) compared to other rices, accounts for its lower G.I. value.
Brown rice	55 (av)	Also called whole rice. It is the whole grain with the fibrous inedible outer hull removed. This nutty-flavored rice, long or medium grain, is the most nutritious form of rice.
Uncle Ben's Converted	44	This highly nutritious rice is the same as parboiled. In the parboiling process, water-soluble nutrients are transferred from the germ and outer layers to the interior.
Instant	87	One brand of instant rice is Minute Rice, which has been pre-cooked to shorten its preparation time. It's more expensive and less nutritious than the other forms of white rice.
Long grain white	56	These rice grains remain separate when cooked and will only become sticky if they're overcooked or over stirred. One grain measures at least one-quarter inch.
Short grain Japanese rice	48	This short grain rice, which is eaten by people every day in Japan, has a low glycemic index despite an amylose content of only 20 percent.
Waxy rice (0–2 percent amylose)	88	This sticky rice is used in rice desserts; it has a very high glycemic index, probably due to the absence of amylose starch.

THE GI VALUES OF NOODLES

PRODUCT	G.I.	COMMENT
Vermicelli	35	A thinner version of spaghetti that cooks quickly and is great added to soups and stir-fries.
Lungkow bean thread noodles	26	Also known as cellophane noodles or green bean vermicelli, these shiny fine white noodles are made from mung beans. Their low glycemic index comes from their legume origin and noodle shape. Soak them in hot water then add to stir-fries and salads. Look for them in Asian supermarkets.
Instant noodles	47	You'll find these noodles in some dehydrated soups that, when reconstituted and heated for a very short time, are completely cooked. The nutritional downside of this popular food is that it is generally high in fat and sodium.

The Take Home Message

- Traditional Asian-style diets, characterized by large amounts of rice and small amounts of meat, offer many health benefits.
- Eat low G.I. rices.
- Choose rice noodles in place of high G.I. rice.
- Eat seven servings of fruit and vegetables a day.
- Choose large servings of soy products, such as tofu, miso, soy milk, tempeh and roasted soy nuts.

glucose revolution life plan
asian-style menu

Breakfast
Almond-peach soy milk smoothie

Snack
Large apple or pear

Lunch
Low G.I. boiled rice
Shrimp chow mein
Steamed broccoli with garlic sauce
Fortune cookies

Dinner
Warmed sesame noodles
Marinated flank steak strips
Frozen stir-fry vegetables
Large tossed salad
Berries or seasonal fruit salad

Snack
Chocolate- or vanilla-flavored soy milk

CHAPTER 6

Paleolithic Nutrition:
The High Protein Diet

HUMANS HAVE COME a long way since prehistoric days of hunting and gathering. Almost everything has changed, including our diets! But one thing has remained basically unaltered: our genes. About 99 percent of our genetic make-up was defined long before our forebears evolved into Homo sapiens some 50,000 years ago. Scientists believe that about seven million years ago, one chimpanzee species began the gradual process of human evolution. The first human-like creatures walked upright about four million years ago; then, about $2\frac{1}{2}$ million years ago the climate in Africa and elsewhere began to cool down, causing what was to be the first of a long series of ice ages. Rainforests eventually gave way to savanna; grassland became the dominant vegetation. In this new climate, herbivorous (plant-eating) animals proliferated, as did the carnivorous (meat-eating) creatures that preyed upon them.

The last two million years of human evolution have occurred against a backdrop of ice ages, spiked by short, warmer interglacial periods, such as we're in now. As you might imagine, vegetation on the planet is markedly different during an ice age: More water becomes locked in the polar ice caps, there is less rainfall and, as a result, less plant growth. These climate changes had important implications for animals; to survive, they adapted and adjusted to the new food chain, and humans became increasingly carnivorous.

how we have evolved metabolically

Metabolically, we are a product of these two million years of evolution and have a great deal in common with meat-eating animals. For example, our bodies need a good amount of iron, iodine and zinc, and we only have a limited ability to synthesize the essential fatty acids, vitamin A and the amino acid taurine. Not coincidentally, animal foods are the best sources of these nutrients.

Our guts are significantly smaller and our brains markedly bigger than those of other primates. Our energy-demanding brains could only have come about if our guts became less demanding and our food more con-centrated, which is known as the "expensive brain hypothesis." What does this mean for current dietary recommendations? For far too long we've assumed that humans adapt quickly and readily to radical dietary changes. In fact, our genes are *still* equipped for the Ice Ages, not the current warm period in which agriculture dominates. In other words, our genes—and our metabolism—are programmed for nutrient intake within a well-defined range: We can't exist on the diet of our simian ancestors (leaves, fruit and berries), made most clearly evident in our essential requirement for vitamin B_{12}, which comes only from animal foods. Just as you would not expect a cat (a true carnivore) to eat grains and fruit, or a giraffe to eat meat, it may be too much to expect that we humans will get away with eat-ing a diet that is too far removed from what we ate as Stone Age people.

During the past two million years of human evolution—except for the last 10,000 years when agriculture was developing—we have been hunter-gatherers rather than farmers. The advent of agriculture is critical because when we started growing crops, particularly cereal grains, we started eat-ing a lot more starch, tipping the ratio of animal to plant foods from being more animal to more plant. And the ratio of the major nutrients changed radically, too. It's a misconception that our evolutionary diet was a kind of vegetarian diet—that's true if you go back a long, long way, but it is not true of the species that evolved into Homo sapiens.

So maybe it's time to look more carefully at our ancestors' eating habits as a guide to the best diet for optimum health: Prehistoric hunting for meat and foraging for vegetables may well have provided the optimum exercise and dietary regime for human survival! In fact, now that we're eating higher carbohydrate and lower protein diets, we may be eating less animal food (meat, seafood, eggs) than our bodies were designed for. Keep in mind that the higher protein diets we're talking about refer to the Paleolithic diet, *not* the high protein diets being touted in the media today. Although the Paleolithic diet was more protein- than carbohydrate-based, the protein came from lean meats and legumes, and the carbohydrates were unrefined, so these diets most probably had low G.I. values In fact, these diets have much in common with the Glucose Revolution Life Plan, because we also recommend eating fruits, vegetables, grains, nuts and some lean meat.

the prehistoric larder

There's little doubt that our Stone Age cousins ate a diet that's very different than the one we eat today. Experts once estimated that the daily nutrient intake of our Paleolithic ancestors consisted of a diet of 65 percent plant food and 35 percent animal sources. It now seems likely, however, that those numbers were completely the opposite of what experts now estimate. In fact, a new analysis shows that the average ratio of plant to animal foods (by energy, or calories) was just the opposite: 65 percent *animal* food, 35 percent *plant* foods. Experts have also reported that our prehistoric relatives consumed exceedingly high levels of fiber. Fruit, roots, legumes and nuts provided the Paleolithic forager with 100 grams of fiber a day, which stands in sharp contrast to the current recommendations of 30 grams a day. The health advantages of their high fiber diet would have been considerable: Indeed, our ancestors would have had low rates of diabetes, colon cancer and anemia.

carbohydrates before agriculture

Carbohydrate levels in prehistoric diets were lower than current recommended levels (see "Comparative Diets: Then and Now" on page 71). But, before the agricultural age, carbohydrates were derived almost exclusively from nuts, legumes, fruit and vegetables. So all the carbohydrates that our ancestors ate would have had a low glycemic index.

In addition to eating more cancer-fighting fruits and vegetables, our ancestors ate more slowly digestible carbohydrates, too. These dietary changes may help to explain why some people, such as Native Americans, who have gone directly from hunter–gatherer diets to meals focusing on more highly-digestible carbohydrates, currently suffer such high rates of diabetes and heart disease.

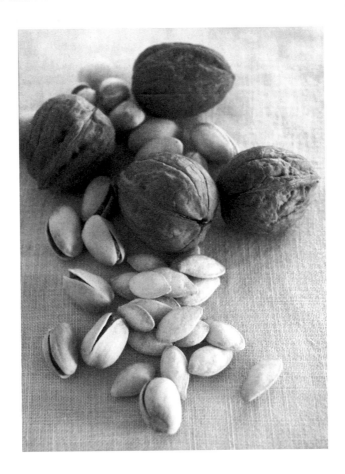

Paleolithic Versus Contemporary Nutrient Intake

	PALEOLITHIC	CURRENT
VITAMINS		
Riboflavin	6.5	1.7
Folate	0.36	0.18
Thiamin	3.9	1.5
Ascorbate	600	60
Vitamin A	17	6
Vitamin E	33	10
	PALEOLITHIC	CURRENT
MINERALS		
Iron	87	10–15
Zinc	43	15
Calcium	1,950	800–1,200
Sodium	770	500–2,400
Potassium	10,500	3,500

The estimated daily Paleolithic intake (milligrams per day) of selected nutrients compared to current recommended levels (from Boyd Eaton et al., *New England Journal of Medicine*, 1985)

═══ Comparative Diets: Then And Now ═══

	PALEOLITHIC	CURRENT DIETARY GUIDELINES
Protein	20–40%	15%
Carbohydrate	20%	55%
Fat	40–60%	30%

Cordain L., Brand-Miller, J., Eaton, S. B., Mann, N., "Plant-Animal Subsistence Ratios and Macronutrient Energy Estimations in Worldwide Hunter-Gatherer Diets," *American Journal of Clinical Nutrition*, 71 (3): 682-92, 2000.

the mammoth eaters

The most significant difference between prehistoric and late-20th-century diets is in the amount of protein consumed (see "Comparative Diets: Then and Now" on page 71). There is overwhelming evidence to suggest that Paleolithic humans consumed large amounts of meat (a type of meat, by the way, that had nothing in common with the saturated-fat-laden grain-fed livestock that provides the meats that we eat today). Evidence suggests that the game meat our prehistoric ancestors ate was low in saturated fats.

Although prehistoric hunters consumed vast amounts of cholesterol—480 milligrams (mg.) daily, according to researchers—experts estimate that their blood cholesterol levels were much lower than today's cholesterol levels. Why? We know by analyzing Paleolithic diets that our prehistoric ancestors ate nearly equivalent amounts of omega-3 and omega-6 fats, which bestowed great health benefits: Eating more protein without saturated fats would have improved our ancestors' blood lipid profiles. In particular, their "good" HDL cholesterol would have been higher, so the risk of chronic heart disease would probably have been lower.

Although we tend to associate meat-eating with an increased risk of cancer and heart disease, that's something of a simplification. We run into trouble when the meat we eat is high in fat and when we don't eat enough fruits and vegetables. Unfortunately, this is actually how most of us now eat, which may explain the rising incidence of obesity, diabetes and heart disease in America.

diet and survival

The evidence suggests that our genetic heritage was shaped over millions of years by a successful combination of animal foods, fruit and vegetables. Today, we substitute some of these foods with dairy products and grain foods, neither of which were significant food sources in hunter-gatherer diets. Paleolithic peoples had little need for today's gourmet foods and dietary supplements, because their intake of essential minerals and vitamins, especially sources of vitamin C, were extraordinarily high (see "Paleolithic versus Contemporary Nutrient Intake" on page 71). Even their calcium intake was high, despite the lack of dairy foods. High protein foods such as meat and seafood, which are more filling, combined with large servings of non-cereal plants, would have made for a very satisfying diet.

old ways for new?

We've discussed how our ancestors' diets differed vastly from our own, but the physiology and biochemistry they passed down through the generations is the same. Some nutritionists are now recommending not only a higher fruit and vegetable intake, but also a higher protein and lower carbohydrate diet.

Protein is the most filling of all the nutrients; it also stimulates heat production, which makes weight control easier. Indeed, one recent study showed greater weight and fat loss on a high protein, low fat diet compared with a normal, high carbohydrate-low fat diet. High protein, low fat diets have also been shown to improve HDL and **triglycerides** in the blood, too. (But we're certainly *not* endorsing the high protein fad diets that are currently popular. Remember, those food plans are neither low in fat nor high in fiber and have little in common with the Paleolithic diet of our ancestors. We also don't recommend high protein diets for people with diabetes, in whom kidney function may be impaired.)

These findings need to be confirmed before we can recommend higher protein and lower carbohydrate diets; we can't yet make dietary recommendations based on evolutionary evidence. This perspective may provide valuable insights, though, into our dietary needs and about the relationships between diet and development and diet and chronic disease.

why current high protein diets don't work

Our ancestors ate wild (low fat) game and fish, legumes, nuts and seeds, as well as fruits and vegetables. Their foods were totally unprocessed and unrefined. In other words, their diet was high in protein and fiber and low in fat and low on the glycemic index.

Today's adaptation of our ancestors' high protein diet is, unfortunately, totally inaccurate. A bun-less bacon cheeseburger and small lettuce salad have little in common with a typical Stone Age meal—whether hunted or gathered. Avoiding fruit, beans and vegetables was not the habit of our ancestors; in fact, looking for these most typical (and low G.I.) foods most likely occupied a good deal of their time.

For years the American Dietetic Association, and other groups interested in our country's nutritional health, have been sending out the very clear message: "Diets don't work!" Certainly the current approach to high protein dieting doesn't work, as proven by the lack of substantive research results:

Initial weight loss is water—not fat—loss. Our bodies simply cannot lose 10 or 5 or even 2 pounds of fat in a weekend, as some testimonials might suggest. The loss is merely water, due to a temporary sodium imbalance, and it will eventually be replenished.

Highly restrictive eating plans quickly lead to boredom and lack of food enjoyment. This boredom may lead to less eating, which then results in weight loss. This strategy is usually short-lived and many dieters give up their high protein diet efforts.

Consistent low calorie intakes will promote weight loss. Anyone eating less than 1,000 calories a day will lose weight, no matter where those calories come from.

People with diabetes may be compromising the health of their kidneys on a high protein diet. Kidneys filter all particles passing through the blood to purify it. When there's a high concentration of sugar in the blood, the added stress of filtering the waste products of a high protein diet may be just too much for your kidneys to handle.

what does work?

There's no magic bullet for permanent weight loss. But looking at research that has tracked people who have lost weight and maintained it over the long haul, certain characteristics emerge. Weight-loss maintainers:

- have a positive attitude toward changing their diet to improve health;
- possess a willingness to lose weight slowly;
- make lasting changes to their diet and exercise patterns; and
- feel comfortable with, rather than restricted by, dietary changes.

the trick to feeling full

You can feel most satisfied after a meal when the foods are of appropriate nutrient proportions. That's why you should strive for adequate protein, fiber, heart-healthy fats and unprocessed or minimally refined carbohydrates in each of your meals. Lucky for all of us, selecting low G.I. foods makes feeling full easy!

═══ *The Take Home Message* ═══

- Human beings ate a high protein, low carbohydrate diet during evolution.
- On average, two-thirds of their energy came from animal foods.
- The wild animals our prehistoric ancestors ate provided varying amounts of fat (sometimes large quantities) but their saturated fat intake was never high.
- A higher-protein, lower-carbohydrate diet that's low in fat and high in fiber may offer benefits today. But people with diabetes should avoid large quantities of protein until we know more about the effect on renal disease.

---

glucose revolution life plan
paleolithic menu

The following menu derives equal proportions of energy from carbohydrate, protein and fat, which we believe may be similar to the diet of humans thousands of years ago. All the sources of carbohydrate in this menu are slowly digested, low G.I. types.

Note: For the menus below, follow the portion sizes listed in "What is a Serving?" on page 83.

Breakfast
Fruit and nut muesli with apple and yogurt
Large apple
Low fat plain yogurt

Lunch and snacks
Open roast beef sandwich (on low G.I. bread)
Large pear
Tuna and egg salad
Mixed bean salad
Trail mix

Dinner
Grilled fish with lemon
Pinto beans
Steamed broccoli, carrot and cabbage
Peaches and strawberries served with ricotta cheese and honey

Part Two

putting the
GLUCOSE
REVOLUTION
LIFE PLAN
into action

CHAPTER 7

The Glucose Revolution Life Plan Eating Style

WE'VE DEVOTED THIS section of the book to the practical details of the Glucose Revolution Life Plan eating style. In Part One we discussed five key areas of current nutrition research: the glycemic index, omega-3 fats, Mediterranean diets, Asian diets and Paleolithic nutrition. As you now know, we believe that certain aspects of these eating styles hold the key to better health.

Now, we're bringing together all of the messages in Part One to present you with the whole plate—a plate that incorporates low G.I. carbohydrate with healthy fats, lean and nutritious sources of protein and phytochemical-rich fruits and vegetables.

components of a healthy diet

A nutritious diet is based on a wide variety of foods, but *not* on a wide variety of fast foods and foods with empty calories! Eat these foods every day:

- Fresh vegetables, cooked and raw
- Fresh fruit
- Whole grain bread and cereals
- Nonfat or low fat milk and part-skim cheese
- Fish, lean meat, chicken, legumes and soy

In addition, you should eat the following foods regularly (but not necessarily daily) and in moderation. These foods are rich in antioxidants, vitamins and minerals, and some of them, such as vinegar, have a specific effect on lowering the glycemic response to carbohydrate. Others, such as nuts, olive oil and avocado, are rich in heart-healthy fats:

- Nuts and seeds
- Olive, canola, peanut oils
- Avocado, olives
- Dried fruit
- Vinegar (vinaigrette for salads)
- Red wine
- Fresh herbs and spices
- Shellfish and other seafood
- Soy products

The table below shows how you could add various protein foods and whole grains to your meals during the week: We encourage you to include fish once or twice a week and legumes at least twice weekly. We include cooked vegetables or salad in all meals and recommend fruit for dessert.

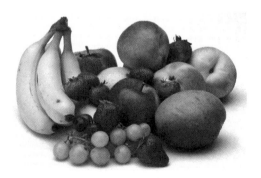

PUTTING TOGETHER MEALS FOR THE WEEK

▶ Lunch: whole grain breads and cereals, low fat proteins, vegetables and salads, fruit and nonfat or low fat dairy foods

▶ Dinner: whole grains, low fat proteins, vegetables and salads, fruit

Examples for the week

	LUNCH	DINNER
MONDAY	Veggie burger	Minestrone soup
TUESDAY	Grilled chicken salad with whole grain bread	Grilled fish with spicy couscous
WEDNESDAY	Lentil or split-pea soup	Lamb or beef stew with barley pilaf
THURSDAY	Hummus on toasted pita bread	Omelet with crusty semolina bread and salad
FRIDAY	Pasta primavera with shrimp	Chicken and broccoli stir fry
SATURDAY	Melted reduced-fat cheese whole grain toast	Pork tenderloin and polenta with mushroom gravy
SUNDAY	Salmon or crab cake	Pan-roasted vegetables with roast beef

1. eat 3 or more servings of fruit and 4 or more servings of vegetables every day

Fruit and vegetables are a major part of low G.I. eating. The greater the variety you eat, the better. Forget dinner plates full of plain boiled vegetables, salads of lettuce and tomato and the daily apple or orange: The variety of fruit and vegetables that we're talking about extends far beyond this!

Specifically, aim to eat four or more servings of vegetables and three servings of fruit every day. Include green vegetables, particularly green leafy vegetables. Choose among broccoli, spinach, green beans, cauliflower, Brussels sprouts, leeks, cabbage, peppers, kale, bok choy. You can eat vegetables steamed or seasoned with fresh or dried herbs, or with a dressing made from olive oil, lemon juice, balsamic vinegar and garlic.

What Is A Serving?

Bread/cereal group

1 slice bread

1 tortilla

1/2 cup cooked rice, pasta or cooked cereal

1 oz. ready-to-eat cereal

2 medium cookies

3–4 small crackers

1 4-inch pancake

Vegetable group

1/2 cup chopped raw or cooked vegetables

1 cup raw leafy vegetables

3/4 cup (6 ozs.) vegetable juice

1/2 cup cooked potatoes

10 French fries

Fruit group

1 medium-size piece fruit

1/2 cup chopped, cooked or canned fruit

1 melon wedge

1/4 cup dried fruit

Dairy group

1 cup (8 ozs.) milk or yogurt

1 1/2 ozs. natural cheese

2 ozs. processed cheese

1 1/2 cups ice cream (regular or reduced fat)

1 cup frozen yogurt

What Is A Serving?

Protein group

2½–3 ozs. cooked red meat, poultry or fish

½ cup cooked beans

1 egg (equal to 1 oz. meat)

2 Tbsp. peanut butter (equal to 1 oz. meat)

⅓ cup nuts (equal to 1 oz. meat)

Fats, oils, sweets group

Use sparingly.

Adapted from the Food Guide Pyramid, Home and Garden Bulletin Number 252, U.S. Department of Agriculture Human Nutrition Information Service.

Eat a salad daily. If you or your children don't enjoy salads very much, try serving it first to catch their appetites when they're most voracious. Try a tossed salad of mixed salad greens, tomatoes, cucumber, red onion, chickpeas and sliced mushrooms. You can even add fruit or nuts if you want. Mix up a large salad at the start of the weekend so you have it on hand for easy meals.

We Americans tend to overlook the natural sweetness of fruit as a perfect finale to our meals (all three of them!) or a quick pick-me-up snack. Fruits are widely available, inexpensive and easy to eat—just like other snack foods—without the added fat and sugar.

Fruit and vegetables have consistently been linked with protection from certain types of cancer. They also contain heart-healthy nutrients including unsaturated oils, fiber, vitamin B_6, folate and vitamin E, which reduce our risk of heart disease. Eating more vegetables, especially salad and tomatoes, decreases the risk of prostate cancer.

easy ways to eat more vegetables

Getting more vegetables into your diet is easier than you think. Here's how to make every meal and snack extra-nutritious:

- Add extra vegetables (frozen are easy) to stir-fried meat, chicken, shrimp, fish or tofu.
- Chop up leftover vegetables, heat and use as omelet filling.
- Try stuffed vegetables—an extraordinary meal. See our recipe for Stuffed Eggplant on page 178.
- Include salad ingredients in a pocket sandwich or tortilla wrap.
- Throw some veggies onto the grill with meat. Try zucchini, corn, peppers, mushrooms, eggplant or thick slices of parboiled sweet potato or onion. (Use vegetable spray on a cold grill or a little olive oil to prevent sticking.)
- Drink low-sodium vegetable juices.
- Try a vegetarian main dish at least once a week. (This is what the American Heart Association recommends.)
- Add grated carrot and zucchini to quick breads and muffins.
- Choose take-out meals that include vegetables. Here are a few choices:
  - ▶ regular hamburger with salad
  - ▶ vegetarian chili
  - ▶ vegetable stir fry
  - ▶ salad sandwiches or rolls
  - ▶ pasta with a tomato-based sauce
  - ▶ vegetable pizza
  - ▶ stuffed potato with beans, salsa and cheese
  - ▶ a side order of salad
  - ▶ meat and vegetable fajitas
- For quick munching, keep celery, peppers, baby carrots, cucumbers, jicama, broccoli or cauliflower florets and cherry or grape tomatoes on hand. Dip them in low fat dip or salsa.
- Try vegetarian lasagna.
- Every week, try a vegetable that you haven't eaten before.

BUYING

Choose veggies that are brightly colored, bruise-free and not wilted. They taste best when they're very fresh, so it's best to shop two or three times a week and use produce within two to three days of purchase.

STORING

Loosen bunched vegetables, remove plastic wraps and store loosely in the crisper.

PREPARING

You must wash, then rinse, all vegetables well to remove any fine soil or grit. Many supermarkets and health food stores sell special fruit and vegetable washes, which are liquid solutions designed to remove chemical residue (including pesticides, dirt and oil) from the produce's surface. Green leaves for a salad should be torn into small pieces rather than cut. Use a salad spinner or a clean towel to remove as much water as possible.

Spinach: Shred or chop this green to use in soups, casseroles, omelets, lasagna or stuffing.

Kale, collard, mustard or beet greens, escarole, cabbage: These greens are best cooked with a minimum of water (ideally in a steamer) for three to five minutes. You can also microwave them with just the water that clings to the leaves. Be sure to use only glass or microwaveable plastic containers.

Sweet potato: Boil, steam or microwave potatoes until tender, remove the skin, then mash for soups or casseroles; grill unskinned and slice for a side dish.

Tomatoes: Slice them for salads or topping for quiches, casseroles or vegetable stratas; dice or chop for sauces, soups, salsas and omelet fillings.

TIPS ON COOKING VEGETABLES

- Don't overcook: Cook them until they're softened but still firm to bite.
- Leave the skins on whenever you can.
- Avoid soaking them in water.
- Cook large pieces rather than coarsely chopped fragments.
- Never add bicarbonate of soda to the cooking water.
- Reduce the amount of water you use and cover the pan.
- Cook them quickly and as close to serving time as possible.
- Use a steaming tray or microwave.

easy ways to eat more fruit

Most people find fruit sweet enough to recommend itself. But if you're having a little trouble getting your daily requirement, try these tips.

- Always include fruit (fresh, canned in fruit juice or dried) in or with low G.I. breakfast cereals.
- Top yogurt with fresh fruit.
- Make fresh fruit smoothies or milkshakes.
- Add fruit to fresh salads (examples: apples, citrus, grapes, strawberries, pears).
- Use fruit salsas in omelets, with fish or pork, as a salad dressing or a chip dip.
- Stew fresh fruit for compotes or for pancake and waffle toppings.
- For a quick lunch, try an apple or pear with some cheese and whole-grain crackers.
- Make your own jam with your favorite in-season fruit.
- Bake, broil, grill or microwave meaty fruits such as apples or pears for a warm dessert.
- Carry a piece of fresh fruit or a few dried apricots to work or when you travel for a quick and readily available snack (one that just happens to be nutritious and low G.I.!).

═══ Enjoy a Kaleidoscope of ═══ Fruits and Vegetables

The world of fruits and vegetables is colorful, indeed! Here are some examples of the wide variety of produce you can enjoy every day.

Green: Salad greens, asparagus, broccoli, celery, cucumber, green beans, kale, peas, peppers, scallions, spinach, apples, figs, honeydew melon, pears

Red: Kidney beans, peppers, pinto beans, radishes, tomatoes, apples, cherries, pears, plums, raspberries, strawberries

White: Cauliflower, cannellini beans, onions

Orange: Carrots, peppers, sweet potato, squash (acorn, butternut), apricots, cantaloupe, nectarines, oranges, peaches, tangerines

Yellow: Corn, spaghetti squash, bananas, grapefruit, pears

Brown: Garbanzo beans, mushrooms, pears

Purple: Eggplant, blackberries, blueberries, figs, plums

TIPS ON BUYING AND USING FRUIT

BUYING

Choose brightly colored, bruise-free fruit; stems shouldn't be black and shriveled. Try to buy fruits with varying degrees of ripeness in order to have ready-to-eat fruit always available.

STORING

You can store your fruit as you prefer: Some people like cold fruit, while others would rather eat it at room temperature. When it comes to fresh fruit, suit yourself. Don't wash it too soon, though; water that remains on the fruit for a period of time may hasten the decaying process. Instead, wash fruit just before you eat it.

PREPARING

Wash all fruit thoroughly with a fruit and vegetable wash or with warm soapy water (even fruits that you'll peel). When possible, leave skin on for more nutrients and fiber. Pare and cut fruit just before using it, leaving slices or chunks as large as possible. You may need to toss certain fruit with lemon juice to prevent discoloration.

- **Peaches, strawberries, apples, pears:** Thinly slice these fruits and place them on toasted bread.
- **Apples:** Core apples, dust them with cinnamon and bake.
- **Peaches, nectarines, pears, plums, apricots:** Halve these fruits, remove the pits and poach them with or without the skin.
- **Figs, peaches, nectarines, pears:** Halve, then coat these fruits with butter, margarine or vegetable spray and grill.

TIPS ON COOKING FRUIT

- Don't overcook fruit. Rule of thumb: The juicier the fruit, the less cooking time required.
- Cook fruit quickly and as close to serving time as possible.
- For best results, use fresh fruit in season.
- If you're trying a new recipe or creating your own, account for cooking shrinkage.
- Avoid using bruised fruit, or if bruising is minimal, cut away all the discolored pulp.
- Never cook moldy fruit; throw it away.
- Consider the best degree of ripeness for your recipe.

2. eat wholegrain breads and cereals with a low glycemic index

Cereal grains including rice, wheat, oats, barley, rye and products made from them (including bread, pasta, breakfast cereal and flours) are the most concentrated sources of carbohydrate in our diet, with carbohydrate amounts ranging from 50 to 80 percent of their weight. (Compare this to the carbohydrate content of fruit—around 10 to 15 percent—and root vegetables such as potato—around 15 to 20 percent.) Because of the significant amount of carbohydrate in cereal grains, they have a major impact on the glycemic index of our diet.

Some people might argue that the demise of the human diet began with the industrial revolution and the refining of cereal grains. Traditionally, preparing grains was simple, limited to grinding the grains between stones. So, for the most part, grains kept their original form, which meant they were slowly digested and absorbed. Our ancestors ate most of their carbohydrate like this, including fruits, vegetables, beans and whole cereal grains—all sources of carbohydrate with low G.I. values.

The advent of high-speed steel roller mills in the 19th century made the production of fine white flours and their derivatives—such as soft breads, cakes, doughnuts and corn flakes—possible. Our modern Western diet tends to be based on these quickly digested carbohydrates, which results in much greater rises in blood sugar and insulin levels than most of our bodies have evolved to cope with. As a result, many of us now suffer from diseases such as diabetes, heart disease and obesity in epidemic proportions.

So significant is the health impact of the glycemic index that the WHO/FAO now recommends that we should choose foods with a low glycemic index. For these reasons, we think that low G.I. breads and cereals are a crucial part of healthy eating.

Choose breads and cereals with a low glycemic index such as:

- low G.I. breakfast cereals (based on wheat bran, psyllium and oats);
- grainy breads made with barley, rye, linseed, triticale (a wheat and rye hybrid), sunflower seed, oats, soy and cracked wheat;
- pasta products in place of potatoes; and
- low G.I. rices such as long grain white rice, brown rice.

Not only do whole grains have a lower glycemic index than refined cereal grains but also they are nutritionally superior, containing higher levels of fiber, vitamins, minerals and phytochemicals. Studies show that higher consumption of whole grains is associated with reduced incidence of cancer and heart disease. A large survey of post-menopausal women showed a clear relationship between their intake of whole grains and risk of death from some forms of heart disease: In fact, the risk of dying from heart disease was reduced by about one-third in those women eating one or more servings of whole grain product each day.

	G.I. VALUE
Low G.I breakfast cereals	
All Bran with Extra Fiber	51
Bran Buds with Psyllium	45
Muesli, natural	56
Muesli, toasted	43
Oatmeal, old-fashioned	42
Special K	54
Low G.I. breads	
Pita, whole wheat	57
Pumpernickel, whole grain	51
Sourdough	52
Sourdough rye	57
Whole wheat, 100% stoneground	53
Low G.I. cereal grains	
Barley	25
Buckwheat	54
Bulgur	48
Corn, sweet	55
Rice	
Basmati	58
Brown	55
Uncle Ben's converted	44
White, long-grain	56

more about cereals and grains

BARLEY
G.I. VALUE: 25

One of the oldest cultivated cereals, barley is very nutritious and high in soluble fiber, which helps to reduce the post-meal rise in blood glucose and lowers its glycemic index. Look for products such as pearl barley to use in soups, stews and pilafs, and barley flakes or rolled barley, which have a light, nutty flavor and can be cooked as a cereal and used in baked goods and stuffing.

BULGUR
G.I. VALUE: 48

Also known as cracked wheat, bulgur is made from wheat grains that have been hulled and steamed before grinding to crack the grain. The whole wheat grain in bulgur remains virtually intact—it is simply cracked—and the wheat germ and bran are retained, which preserves nutrients and lowers the glycemic index. Bulgur is used as the base of the Middle Eastern salad tabouli, but can also be used in pilafs, veggie burgers, stuffing, stews, salads and soups or as a cereal.

CORN
G.I. VALUE: 55

Corn is an excellent source of fiber and popular with children. Fresh, frozen and canned varieties of corn have a low glycemic index; products such as corn chips and corn flakes, though, do not.

OATS
G.I. VALUE OF OATMEAL: 42

Rolled oats are whole grain oats that have been hulled, steamed and flattened; this popular cereal grain lowers the glycemic index of oatmeal, granola, cookies, bread and meatloaf. Oat bran also has a low glycemic index.

RICE

G.I. VALUES VARY: SEE TABLE ON PAGE 91.

Rice can have a high G.I. value (80–90) or a low G.I. ranking (50–55) depending on the variety and, in particular, its amylose content. Amylose is a type of starch that we digest more slowly, which gives foods a lower glycemic index. (High amylopectin starch produces a higher glycemic response.) *Brown* (G.I. 55), *Basmati rice* (G.I. 58) and *Uncle Ben's converted rice* (G.I. 44) contain higher proportions of amylose, which produces a lower glycemic response, is more compact in structure and more slowly digested. *Waxy* or *glutinous rice*, which becomes sticky when cooked, has a high glycemic index, and is preferred for rice desserts. *Arborio rice*, which is especially good for making Italian risotto, releases its starch during cooking and is likely to have a high glycemic index as a result. *Japonica rice*, eaten all over Japan, is a short grain variety with a low G.I value.

RYE

G.I. VALUE OF WHOLE KERNEL RYE: 34

Whole kernel rye is used to make certain breads, including pumpernickel and some crispbreads (Scandinavian crackers). Rye flakes are similar to rolled oats; you can eat them as a cooked cereal or sprinkle them over bread before you bake it.

WHEAT

G.I. VALUE OF WHOLE WHEAT KERNELS: 41

Wheat provides a staple food to half the world's population. Soak whole wheat overnight and simmer for about an hour to use as a base for pilaf. Some people enjoy wheat bran as a cooked breakfast cereal. Cream of Wheat is made from very fine semolina; you can use it as a breakfast cereal or in puddings, custards, soufflés and soups.

3. eat more legumes (beans, peas and lentils) and use nuts (in small amounts) more frequently

Legumes, including lentils, chickpeas, cannellini beans, soybeans and kidney beans, are an important part of a low G.I. diet; we suggest that you eat them at least twice a week. You can eat more legumes by including them in soups, salads and sauces.

Legumes are nutrient dense, providing protein, iron, zinc, calcium, folate and soluble fiber. They're also an excellent source of phytoestrogens such as **lignans** and isoflavones. Studies suggest that eating large amounts of foods rich in phytoestrogens can reduce the risk of several diseases: The activity of lignans and isoflavones, for example, may control some menopausal symptoms. What's more, lignans and isoflavones possess antiviral, antifungal, antibacterial and anti-cancer properties. Flavones also have antihypertensive, anti-inflammatory and antioxidant activities. Beans are high in folate, which lowers the level of homocysteine in the blood and reduces the risk of heart disease.

Legumes are:

- inexpensive
- low in calories
- free of saturated fat and cholesterol
- filling

Soybeans are particularly rich in ALA (the plant precursor of omega-3s), and also contain genistein—an anti-cancer phytochemical. Tofu (soy bean curd) is an easy way of using soy. It has a mild flavor itself but absorbs the flavors of other foods, making it delicious when it's been marinated in soy sauce, ginger and garlic and tossed into a stir-fry. Try our recipe for Tofu Chicken with Snow Peas and Rice Noodles on page 175.

Legumes supply carbohydrate and protein but very little fat. They're high in fiber—both soluble and insoluble—and are a great source of vitamins. Although they will keep indefinitely, it's best to use dried legumes within one year of purchase. Young beans cook faster than old ones and will also be more vividly colored.

dried legume preparation

1. **Soak.** Place legumes in a saucepan and cover them with two to three times their volume of cold water. (Soak them overnight or during the day.)

   Shortcut: Rather than soaking overnight, add three times the volume of water to rinsed beans, bring to a boil for a few minutes then remove from heat and let soak for an hour. Drain, add fresh water then cook as usual.

2. **Cook.** Drain off the soaking water, adding two to three times the volume of water as beans. Bring the water to a boil then simmer until beans are tender. Use the directions on the packet or the information below as a time guide.

   - Don't add salt to the cooking water—it slows down water absorption so cooking takes longer.
   - Don't cook beans in the water they have soaked in. Substances that contribute to flatulence are leached from the beans into the soaking and cooking waters.

Shortcuts: Precooked canned legumes make cooking with beans quick and easy. Legume-based meals come together much faster than those based on meat.

- Precook your own dried legumes and freeze them in small batches.
- You can keep soaked or cooked beans in an airtight container for several days in the fridge.
- One 15.5-oz. can of beans substitutes for ¾ cup of dried beans.

some varieties of beans

CHICKPEAS (ALSO KNOWN AS GARBANZO BEANS)
G.I. VALUE OF BOILED BEANS: 33
G.I. VALUE OF CANNED BEANS: 42

These large, caramel-colored legumes are popular in Middle Eastern and Mediterranean dishes. You can buy them in cans or as dried beans in 1-pound plastic bags. To cook chickpeas, place them in a bowl, cover them with plenty of cold water and soak them overnight. Drain the water, then put the chickpeas in a saucepan and cover them with clean water. Bring the beans to a boil for 10 minutes then simmer for 1½ hours until they're tender to bite. Ground chickpea flour (also called gram flour, or baisen) is used to make unleavened Indian bread; you can also roast and salt whole chickpeas for a delicious snack food.

RED KIDNEY BEANS
G.I. VALUE OF BOILED BEANS: 27
G.I. VALUE OF CANNED BEANS: 52

These are the red beans you find in Mexican dishes such as chili con carne, nachos and tacos. Soak dried beans overnight, then drain and rinse them. Add fresh water, boil 15 minutes then simmer 1 to 1½ hours. After you drain and rinse them, you can use canned kidney beans in soups and salads.

SPLIT PEAS
G.I. VALUE OF BOILED YELLOW PEAS: 32

Green or yellow split peas are a great addition to soups and will cook in about 40 minutes without pre-soaking. Green split peas are traditionally used in pea and ham soups.

LENTILS
G.I. VALUE OF BOILED GREEN AND BROWN LENTILS: 30
G.I. VALUE OF BOILED RED LENTILS: 26

Lentils are available as either whole or split, and are relatively quick cooking, needing to simmer, partly covered for only 10 to 15 minutes, without pre-soaking. You need to boil dried whole lentils, sold in 1-pound plastic bags, for about 45 minutes.

CANNELLINI BEANS
G.I. VALUE: 31

These small, mildly-flavored white beans, highly prized in Italy, are available dried or in cans. Dried beans need to be soaked overnight. Drain, then rinse and add fresh water. Boil for 15 minutes and then simmer for 1 to $1\frac{1}{2}$ hours to make them tender.

MAKING THE MOST OF NUTS

In a Mediterranean diet, people eat nuts and seeds (including almonds, walnuts, pumpkin and sunflower seeds, tahini and roasted chickpeas) once or twice a week. Research suggests that eating a small handful of nuts (1 ounce) several times a week can help lower cholesterol and reduce heart attack risk. Nuts are healthy because they contain:

- very little saturated fat (the fats are predominantly mono- or polyunsaturated)
- dietary fiber
- vitamin E, an antioxidant believed to help prevent heart disease

Walnuts and pecans also contain some omega-3 fats, while linseeds are very rich in omega-3s, lignans and plant estrogens. When freshly ground, linseeds have a subtle nutty flavor and make a great addition to breads, muffins, biscuits and cereals.

EASY WAYS TO EAT MORE NUTS

- Use nuts and seeds in food preparation: for example, use toasted cashews or sesame seeds in a chicken stir-fry, sprinkle walnuts or pine nuts over a salad, top fruity desserts or granola with almonds.
- Spread bread with peanut, almond or cashew butter rather than butter or margarine.
- Sprinkle a mixture of ground nuts and linseeds over cereal or salads, or add to baked goods such as muffins.
- Enjoy nuts as a snack. Although high in fat, nuts make a healthy sub-

stitute for less nutritious high fat snacks such as potato chips, chocolate and cookies.

4. eat more fish and seafood

In studies, weekly fish consumption is linked to a reduced risk of coronary heart disease. In fact, just one serving of fish a week may reduce the
risk of a fatal heart attack by 40 percent. The likely protective components of fish are the very long chain omega-3 fatty acids: eicosapentanoic
acid (EPA) and docosahexanoic acid (DHA). Our bodies only make small
amounts of these fatty acids and so we rely on dietary sources, especially
fish and seafood, for them. (See Chapter 3 for more on the benefits of
omega-3 fats.) The American Heart Association recommends that
American adults eat fish at least twice a week.

Just remember not to cook your fish in solid (saturated) fat. That means
that eating fried fish from a fast-food restaurant doesn't count, nor does
eating pre-cooked breaded frozen-fish products that have been cooked in
saturated oils.

WHICH FISH IS BEST?

Oily fish, which tend to have darker colored flesh and a stronger fishy flavor, are the richest source of omega-3 fats. (Don't be put off by the term
"fatty" or "oily" fish: four ounces of the fattiest fish has about the same
amount of fat as four ounces of very lean beef.)

Canned salmon, sardines, mackerel and, to a lesser extent, tuna, are all
very rich sources of omega-3s; look for canned fish packed in water or soybean, canola or olive oil.

Fresh fish with higher levels of omega-3s are: Atlantic salmon and
smoked salmon, Atlantic, Pacific and Spanish mackerel, sea mullet,
Southern bluefin tuna and swordfish. Eastern and Pacific oysters and
squid (calamari) are also rich sources.

"BUT I DON'T LIKE SEAFOOD!"

If you don't like fish or seafood you'll get some omega-3 fatty acids when you eat lean red meat. If you don't want to eat meat, you can also get a precursor of these fatty acids from plants. This precursor is also an omega-3 fat known as alpha-linolenic acid (ALA). Our bodies can convert this plant-based omega-3 fat to EPA and DHA, but it takes about 10 grams of ALA to yield 1 gram of DHA and EPA. You can get ALA from linseed, canola, walnut and soybean oils. There are also small amounts in walnuts, linseeds, pecans, soybeans, baked beans, wheat germ, lean meats, and green leafy vegetables.

You can also include more omega-3s in your diet by taking fish oil supplements, but it's unlikely that you would get the full benefit of increased omega-3 intake without changing your lifestyle in other ways as well, including getting more exercise, eating a high fiber, low fat balanced diet and quitting smoking. (A supplement, no matter how helpful, can't substitute for a healthy diet and good exercise habits.) Choose a product with the largest amount of EPA and DHA. But be careful—in a 1,000-milligram capsule the amount of EPA and DHA can vary considerably. Look for a product that includes vitamin E, which will help prevent the fish oils from oxidizing.

IS COD LIVER OIL A SOURCE OF OMEGA-3 FATTY ACIDS?

Although cod liver oil contains some omega-3 fats, the amounts are quite small. But it does contain a lot of vitamins A and D, two fat-soluble vitamins that our bodies store. If you were to take enough cod liver oil to meet your omega-3 requirement, you'd also exceed the recommended intake of vitamins A and D.

5. eat lean meats and low fat dairy foods

Eating lean meats and low fat dairy foods is a great way to lower the saturated fat content of your diet. Scientists have known for years that a diet high in saturated fat raises cholesterol levels and increases heart disease risk. More recently, research has also implicated these fats in both insulin resistance and obesity: We burn saturated fat more poorly than other fats, so it tends to be stored as fat more readily. In contrast, our bodies are more likely to use omega-3 PUFAs and MUFAs for energy rather than storage.

Saturated fats should comprise less than 10 percent of our total calorie intake: For an average adult eating around 1800 to 2100 calories, this means eating about 20 grams of saturated fat a day. Unfortunately, the message to "avoid saturated fat" has, for many people, translated into "avoid red meat and dairy products," removing primary sources of iron and calcium from their diets. While it is true that these two food groups could contribute saturated fat to our diets, avoiding these foods entirely will not result in a healthier way of eating.

We suggest eating lean meat two or three times a week, and accompanying it with salad and vegetables. Trim all visible fat from meat, especially pork, and remove the skin (and the fat just below it) from chicken. Game meat such as rabbit and venison are not only lean but are also good sources of omega-3 fatty acids, as are organ meats such as liver and kidney. Replacing full fat dairy foods with reduced fat, low fat or fat free varieties will also help you reduce your saturated fat intake.

Much of the saturated fat we consume these days comes from pre-prepared packaged and take-out foods; in fact, many fast-food restaurants cook with highly saturated fat. Until these restaurants make an effort to reduce the saturated fat content of their products, it's best to eat as little fried fast food as possible.

THE PLACE FOR EGGS AND OTHER CHOLESTEROL-RICH FOODS

We used to think that eating high cholesterol foods such as eggs, shrimp, and other crustaceans would raise our blood cholesterol levels. We now know that our livers compensate for the increased cholesterol intake by reducing cholesterol production (although a small percentage of people have an inherited condition called *familial hypercholesterolemia*, which impairs this self-regulation). This means that you could eat an egg a day, for example, without harming your heart. To enhance your intake of omega-3 fats we suggest that you eat omega-3 enriched eggs (if you can find them), which have about six times more ALA and DHA than regular eggs. These enriched eggs are produced by feeding hens a diet that is naturally rich in omega-3s (including canola and linseeds).

FOODS HIGH IN SATURATED FAT

FOOD TYPE	SATURATED FAT CONTENT (G)
Corn chips (1 oz. bag)	1
Shortening (1 tablespoon)	2
Potato chips (1 oz. bag)	3
Chicken nuggets (6)	3
Doughnut, jelly	4
Medium chocolate shake	4
Chili hot dog	5
Oreo cookies, 3	5
Ice cream, vanilla (2 scoops)	5
Fried chicken, KFC (thigh)	6
Whole milk (1 cup)	6
Croissant	7
Whipped cream (2 Tbsp)	7
Sausage (1)	8
Butter (1 tablespoon)	8
Large French fries	9
Beef burrito (1)	11
Whopper	11
Cheese, American (2 ozs.)	11
Pizza with pepperoni and cheese toppings (2 slices)	14
Burger King BK chicken sandwich	26

6. use high omega-3 and monounsaturated oils such as olive, peanut and canola oils

The following oils are rich in monounsaturated fatty acids, which should supply the majority of fat in our diets.

Olive oil has been a part of the Mediterranean and Middle Eastern diet for thousands of years, and is recognized as a healthy alternative to other fats and oils because it's high in monounsaturated fats and low in saturates. Its minimal PUFA content is also an advantage because it allows our bodies to make greater use of the omega-3 fats we obtain from other dietary sources, without any competition from excessive polyunsaturated omega-6 fats. (See pages 98-99 for more details.) Olive oil has other virtues, too: It's rich in antioxidants and an anti-inflammatory substance called **squalene**, slows blood clot formation and lowers cholesterol.

Peanut oil is a multi-purpose, mild-tasting oil that oxidizes slowly and can withstand high cooking temperatures. About 50 percent of the fat in peanut oil is monounsaturated and another 30 percent is polyunsaturated. This heart-healthy fat is frequently used in Asian cooking.

Canola oil, besides being high in monounsaturated fat, canola contains significant amounts of alpha-linolenic acid (ALA), the plant form of polyunsaturated omega-3 fat. (Canola oil contains approximately 2 grams of ALA per tablespoon.) You can buy margarines made from canola and olive oils in supermarkets; some brand names include: Take Control, Smart Beat, Benecol and Lee Iacocca's Olivio Premium Spread.

Linseed oil is the richest plant source of ALA (one tablespoon provides approximately 9 grams) and it contains very little omega-6 fat. But linseed oil is highly prone to oxidation—meaning the fats it contains turn rancid easily. For this reason, we suggest using linseeds as a source of ALA rather than linseed oil.

Sunola oil is another highly monounsaturated oil. It is a genetic variant of sunflower oil and is very heat stable, making it an ideal alternative to the saturated fats that manufacturers normally use for frying. Like olive oil, sunola oil is omega neutral.

Flaxseed, though not commonly used, is an excellent source of omega-3s. When it's fresh, it tastes sweet and nutty, but it does deteriorate quickly, making it taste unpleasant. Flaxseeds are also loaded with omega-3s. One tablespoon of flaxseed oil or 2 tablespoons of ground flaxseeds daily provide you with an excellent does of omega-3s. In either form, they're a healthful addition to cereals, salads, breads, muffins and cookies.

Cold pressed oils are among those that have undergone minimal processing. Recent research suggests that these oils may be better for our hearts because they are richer in antioxidant compounds called **polyphenols**. "Cold pressed" means that the oil is extracted from the seed, nut or fruit by mechanical pressing only, without heat or solvents. Cold pressed oils have a stronger flavor and color than their regular counterparts, and they're also much richer in vitamin E (a natural preservative present in oils) and other antioxidants. For example, extra-virgin olive oil—the best quality oil made from the first cold pressing of the olives—contains 30 to 40 different antioxidants. It is dark-colored and strong in flavor.

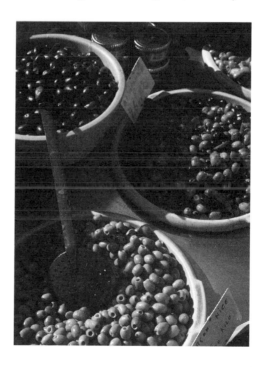

Light and extra light oils are light in color and flavor. The terms "light" and "extra light" don't mean, however, that the oil is lower in fat than any other oil.

Types Of Fat And Their Sources

There is less evidence to support further reducing the amount of fat we eat than there is to recommend changing the type. Although foods contain a mixture of fatty acids, one type of fatty acid tends to predominate, allowing us to categorize foods according to their main fatty acid component.

An asterisk next to a food in the following list means the food is a good source of omega-3 fatty acids.

Polyunsaturated Products

Oils

Safflower, sunflower, grapeseed, soybean*, corn, linseed* (flaxseed), cottonseed, walnut*, sesame, evening primrose oils

Spreads

Polyunsaturated margarines, tahini (sesame seed paste)

Nuts and seeds

Walnuts, sunflower seeds, pumpkin seeds, sesame seeds

Other plant sources

Soybeans, soy milk, wheat germ, whole grains

Animal sources

Oily fish*

Monounsaturated Products

Oils

Olive, canola*, peanut, Sunola™, macadamia and mustard seed oils

Spreads

Monounsaturated margarines made from these oils*, peanut butter

Types Of Fat And Their Sources

Nuts and seeds

Cashews, macadamias, almonds, hazelnuts, pecans, pistachio, peanuts

Other plant sources

Avocado, olives

Animal sources

Very lean red meat, lean chicken, lean pork, egg yolks

Saturated Products

Oils/Fats

Palm and palm kernel oil, coconut oil, drippings, lard, copha, ghee,
   solid frying oils, cooking margarines and shortening

Spreads

Butter, cream cheese

Dairy foods

Full-fat dairy products: cheese, cream, sour cream, yogurt, whole milk,
   ice cream

Animal sources

Fat on beef, lamb, skin on chicken, sausage, salami, most luncheon meats

STORING OLIVE OIL

When storing olive oil, keep the air space in the bottle to a minimum to keep the oil from becoming rancid and store it in a cool, dark place (just don't put it in the refrigerator). Buy only small bottles of oil, or if you buy it in larger amounts, consider decanting it into smaller airtight bottles. Remember, unlike wine, olive oil doesn't improve with age!

VINEGAR

Recent studies have shown that consuming vinegar or lemon juice with a meal can significantly lower blood sugar. As little as one tablespoon of vinegar in a vinaigrette dressing, eaten with an average meal, lowered blood sugar by as much as 30 percent. The effect appears to be related to the food's acidity, which may slow stomach emptying and carbohydrate digestion. Certain studies showed the greatest effect with red wine vinegar and lemon juice, but we've used a range of vinegars in the recipes in this book. Some favorite types of vinegar include:

Balsamic vinegar: Rich and dark, made from sweet wine aged in wooden barrels. It has a sweet, sharp flavor.

Wine vinegar: Made from red or white grapes and popular for salad dressings. It's often flavored with herbs such as tarragon.

Rice wine vinegar: A mild-flavored vinegar distilled from fermented rice.

The Take Home Message

- Eat heart-healthy fats, and foods that contain these fats, more freely.
- Don't go overboard!
- Limit fatty meats and full-fat dairy foods to occasional small portions.
- Avoid commercially prepared foods that contain palm and coconut oils and hydrogenated fat.
- Include: oils, such as olive and canola; lean meats, especially game meat; fish and seafood, including oily fish. Include nuts and seeds.

CHAPTER 8

Get Moving!

DID YOU NOTICE that we used the word "moving," not "exercising?" There's a good reason. Most people think of exercise as a formal and structured activity that they must do each day. Not so! Though some people can and do make a serious commitment to 20 to 30 minutes of exercise three to four times a week, the majority of us say that we're too busy and don't have the time. The result? Many of us make no attempt at all to move our bodies. We're loathe to make *any* effort or commitment: we're too tired, too rushed, too stressed, too hot, too cold—the list of excuses goes on. But there's good news: We don't need to *exercise*, we just need to *move*.

Used to be, experts hinted that unless we exercised vigorously and sustained it for 20 to 30 minutes, we needn't bother doing it in the first place. Now, we know better: Research tells us that any amount of movement is better than none at all. Can you accumulate 30 minutes of moving around each day? We bet you could! Could you weed for say, 5 minutes in the morning, then walk around the neighborhood for 10 minutes later on, then walk up and down the stairs for 2 minutes? That's all it takes to reap important health benefits. And it doesn't need to be vigorous to be beneficial. Nor does it have to involve gyms, special equipment or expensive accessories.

For most people, walking fits the bill perfectly. All of us were meant to walk upright—it's the easiest, safest and most natural form of physical activity around.

walking for pleasure and health

Walking keeps us fit, it's cheap and convenient, and it becomes even more important as we grow older. You can walk alone, or with friends. In fact, talking while you walk can have important emotional benefits: Not only do our bodies produce calming hormones while we walk, but the talk itself can be great therapy—and good for relationships in general. So instead of saying, "How about a cup of coffee?" try, "Would you like to take a walk?" But don't hesitate to walk alone if you prefer, or with your dog—your pet will love you all the more for it. And you'll be able to (finally!) take some time to think and relax.

Walking regularly has scientifically proven benefits. According to the American Heart Association, regular exercise can:

- Help lower blood pressure
- Cut heart attack and diabetes risk
- Reduce insulin requirements if you have diabetes
- Help you stop smoking
- Control weight
- Increase levels of good HDL cholesterol
- Keep bones and joints strong
- Reduce colon cancer risk
- Improve mood
- Ease depression

how often?

Try to walk every day. Ideally you should accumulate 30 minutes or more on most days of the week. The good news is, you can do it in two 15-minute stints or six 5-minute stints. It doesn't matter!

how hard?

You should be able to talk comfortably while you walk. Find a level that suits *you*.

getting started

Before beginning a walking program, see your doctor if you have:

- been inactive for some time
- a history of heart disease or chest pains
- diabetes
- high blood pressure

Or if you:

- weigh more than you should
- smoke

the importance of good shoes

The most important walking equipment is a pair of sturdy, comfortable, lightweight walking shoes. If your feet feel good, you'll want to walk longer distances and stick with your walking program. It's worth the investment!

stop press!

A new study has revealed that greater physical activity is associated with a lower risk of developing type 2 diabetes. Researchers found that the exercise didn't have to be intense: Exercise of moderate duration and intensity—including walking—was associated with reduced risk of disease. While brisk walking was best, even the slow walkers benefited!

10 important tips

Here are a few things to keep in mind as you head out for your next walk.

- Wear a broad-brimmed hat and sunglasses, and use a sunscreen on exposed skin. (Don't forget the tops of your feet if they're exposed.) Avoid the hours between 10 a.m. and 3 p.m. when the sun's rays are strongest. Walk on the shady side of the street.
- Wear well-cushioned flat-soled shoes and layers of clothing that you can remove if you need to.
- Tell someone that you're going for a walk and what time you expect to return.
- Walk steadily. Let your arms swing; get a rhythm going.
- On all your walks, but especially on long or strenuous ones, drink water before you start and carry some with you. A small backpack can carry your water, sunscreen, hat and glasses. Keep it stocked and ready to go.
- If your breathing becomes uncomfortable, slow down. (Don't come to a sudden stop, which can make you dizzy.)
- During the winter wear a hat to keep warm. One-third of our body heat is lost through our heads!
- Avoid walking immediately after meals (wait about 15 minutes), or if you have a fever or bad cold.

- If you're walking in the dark, wear light-colored clothing so that motorists can see you. Carry a flashlight for added visibility.
- If you feel sore at first, don't worry; your body will adapt and the soreness will decrease. Stretching for 2 minutes before and after your walk will help minimize aches and pains.

staying motivated

When we start a new exercise program, we tend to be raring to go! We enjoy being active and nothing can interfere with our routine. But gradually—and often without our even knowing it—we start putting exercise on the back burner. Here are some easy ways to keep physical activity a priority in your life.

- Walk with a regular partner or group.
- Plan your walk in advance: Will it be an early-morning or late-evening stroll?
- Vary your walking location.
- Visit national parks and landmarks.
- Walk your dog (if you have one) at a regular time each day. Soon he'll be reminding you.
- Don't let rain put you off—take your umbrella along and enjoy the sounds.

CHAPTER 9

The Glucose Revolution Life Plan Menus

TO SHOW YOU how the many different aspects of nutrition can fit together to create a low G.I. lifestyle, we've designed some typical healthy menu suggestions. You'll find an emphasis on low G.I. carbohydrates along with plenty of fruit and vegetables, lean meats and seafood and healthy oils.

We've deliberately left quantities off the menus because it is not our intention to prescribe an amount of food to you (particularly considering we don't even know you!). We all have different energy needs and appetites—needs that vary from day to day—and consequently the amount of food we eat may vary from day to day.

If you would like more specific guidance with your diet we suggest you see a Registered Dietitian—check with your local hospital or look in the Yellow Pages under "Dietitians." You can also find a R.D. by calling the American Dietetic Association's Consumer Nutrition Hotline at 800-366-1655 or finding them on the web at www.eatright.org.

If you choose a dietitian on your own, make sure that the person has the letters "R.D." after their name, which indicates that the person has the qualifications and expertise to provide expert nutritional and dietary advice.

```
╔══════════════════════════════════════╗
║      ═══  The Four G.I Menus  ═══      ║
║                                        ║
║   1.  For EveryBody                    ║
║                                        ║
║   2.  For BiggerBodies                 ║
║                                        ║
║   3.  For KidsBodies                   ║
║                                        ║
║   4.  For BusyBodies                   ║
╚══════════════════════════════════════╝
```

There are four different types of menus, with slight modifications according to who will be eating them:

FOR EVERYBODY

These menus are designed for the average adult, and are also suitable for people with type 1 diabetes.

FOR BIGGERBODIES

We've modified these menus for people trying to lose weight, including those with type 2 diabetes. We've emphasized a moderate carbohydrate intake that will satisfy your appetite, with a small amount of fat to save on calories. If appetite isn't a problem you may choose to use the menus for EveryBody, which are slightly higher in fat. Just remember to keep serving sizes in check, or you could gain weight.

FOR KIDSBODIES

We've modified these menus for children. The menus include variations on the dishes in the adult menus, with the inclusion of healthy snacks. Many of the snack foods children eat are high in fat, as well as quickly digested, high G.I. carbohydrate, which may increase their risk of obesity. We suggest some healthier alternatives.

Children are born with a liking for sweet tastes but they also prefer what they're already familiar with. If your kids initially reject a new food, keep trying: They may eventually learn to like new foods if you give them lots of non-threatening opportunities to sample new tastes and textures. A small taste is all it takes, but changes in taste happen gradually, so keep at it!

DRINKS FOR CHILDREN

Offer children water or milk to drink with their meals and limit the amount of juice and soda they have. Four to six ounces is considered one serving of fruit juice; and one to two servings would be an appropriate daily intake. Growing children require three to four 8-ounce glasses of skim or low fat milk a day.

FOR BUSYBODIES

We've modified these menus for very active people. Active people need a high carbohydrate intake to fuel their muscles, but all of the carbohydrates needn't have low G.I. values. So in these menus you'll find large quantities of different types of carbohydrate. We've indicated the G.I. ranking of the carbohydrate in these menus and offer the following tips on when to use high and low G.I. carbohydrates for best performance.

USING THE GLYCEMIC INDEX TO BOOST YOUR SPORTS PERFORMANCE

Scientific research has so far identified three key applications of the glycemic index to enhance sports performance:

1. Use high G.I. foods after exercise, in the recovery phase to enhance glycogen replenishment.
2. Use high G.I. foods or fluids during exercise to maintain blood sugar levels.
3. Eat a low G.I pre-event meal to help enhance endurance in prolonged exercise.

The Best Foods to Include in Your Glucose Revolution Life Plan Menus

Breakfast Foods

Low G.I. fruits

Choose melon, citrus fruits, fresh strawberries, peaches or nectarines, pears, apples, blueberries, raspberries, apricots and grapes. Fruits may be fresh, cooked or packed in water or juice.

Low fat milk

Drink skim or 1 percent milk, or eat light yogurt.

Low G.I. cereals

Good choices include oats, muesli, All Bran with Extra Fiber, oat or rice bran and Special K.

Low G.I. breads

Enjoy wholegrain breads such as 100% stoneground whole wheat, sourdough, sourdough rye, pita and pumpernickel.

Lunch Choices

Vegetables

Savor various salad greens, sprouts, cucumber, tomato, peppers, mushrooms, onions, celery, grated carrot, beetroot, canned corn, shallots, parsley and other fresh herbs.

Low G.I. breads

Try wholegrain breads such as 100% stoneground whole wheat, sourdough, sourdough rye, pita and pumpernickel.

The Best Foods to Include in Your Glucose Revolution Life Plan Menus

Grains

Eat pasta or noodles, rice and cracked wheat for tabouli.

Legumes

Baked beans, canned beans in a salad, lentils or split peas in soup and chickpeas in hummus are all good choices.

Fish

Eat canned tuna, salmon, sardines or crabmeat.

Dairy foods, cheese and milk products

Choose low fat cheeses such as part-skim ricotta or cottage, or look for low fat varieties of American, cheddar or other processed cheeses, feta or goat cheese. Ideal milk choices include skim or 1 percent milk, enriched soy milk, nonfat or low fat yogurt.

Lean meats and other protein foods

Pick ham, chicken breast, turkey or lean roast beef. Peanut butter and tofu are also healthy protein foods.

Fruits

Choose among apples, grapes, pears, oranges, berries, fresh fruit salad, unsweetened canned fruit. When buying fresh, choose fruits in season.

The Best Foods to Include in Your Glucose Revolution Life Plan Menus

Dinner Choices

VEGETABLES

Remember to aim for at least 5 servings a day. Include a large tossed salad every day and eat a wide variety of other vegetables, whether raw or cooked (something green included!).

Starches

Pasta, rice, noodles, couscous, polenta, barley, tortillas and sweet potatoes are all good choices.

Legumes

Enjoy lentils, chickpeas, split peas, kidney beans, pinto beans, black beans, cannellini and baked beans. The American Heart Association recommends that you eat one vegetarian meal each week. Legumes offer lots of variety for vegetarians.

Fish

All fresh and canned fish are good options. Aim for two fish dinners a week, as suggested by the American Heart Association.

Dairy foods, cheese and milk products

Choose low fat cheeses such as part-skim ricotta or cottage, or look for low fat varieties of American, cheddar or other processed cheeses, feta or goat cheese. Ideal milk choices include skim or 1 percent milk, enriched soy milk, nonfat or low fat yogurt.

The Best Foods to Include in Your Glucose Revolution Life Plan Menus

Lean meats

Beef: Choose round cuts (including top round, ground round, bottom round), all loin cuts (such as tenderloin and sirloin), flank, T-bone and Porterhouse steaks.

Pork: Look for center and loin cuts (such as center cut ham pork chops, loin chops, sirloin or tenderloin roast and Canadian bacon).

Lamb: Buy leg, loin chops.

Veal: All cuts make good choices.

Poultry

Enjoy skinless chicken and turkey breast meat.

Fruits

End your meals with fresh fruit—it makes an ideal choice. When fresh fruit isn't available, consider some dried fruits (such as figs, apples, pears and apricots). Also try canned (water or juice packed) and frozen fruits. Good fruit choices include apples, grapes, pears, oranges, berries, fresh fruit salad, unsweetened canned fruit. When buying fresh, choose fruits in season.

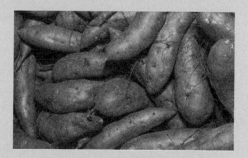

7-day Glucose Revolution
Life Plan Menus

—For Everybody

(an asterisk* next to a meal indicates that the recipe is included in this book.)

Note: For the menus below, follow the portion sizes listed in "What is a Serving?" on page 83.

Monday

Breakfast

100% whole wheat toast
with peanut butter and
apple butter
Fresh orange

Lunch

Minestrone soup
Crusty bread roll
Low fat yogurt and berries

Dinner

Cod fillets with sun-dried
tomato marinade*
Brown rice
Green beans
Mesclun and cherry tomato
salad

Tuesday

Breakfast

Low fat granola topped with
low fat or light yogurt and
sliced berries
Apple juice

Lunch

Mixed Mediterranean salad
(lettuce, tomato, cucumber,
pepppers, olives and beans)
with tomato-olive
vinaigrette*
Pita bread with hummus
A bunch of grapes

Dinner

Grilled basted chicken breast
served with spinach
and snow peas or
corn on the cob

Wednesday

Breakfast

Old-fashioned oatsand low
fat milk flavored with
honey and vanilla
Plate of fresh melon slices
No-sugar-added
hot chocolate

Lunch

Tuna salad served with
lettuce, sliced cucumber,
carrots, tomatoes and
celery with low
G.I. cracker or on
pita bread

Dinner

Vegetable sesame noodle
stir-fry*
Softly simmered
peaches* topped with
light yogurt and a
sprinkle of toasted
walnuts

Thursday

Breakfast

Poached egg and wholegrain
toast with tub margarine
Fresh grapefruit

Lunch

Toasted pita bread with
hummus* and tabouli
Fruit smoothie

Dinner

Pork fillet with spiced pears
and basmati rice*
Steamed carrots and zucchini
(or other fresh vegetable)

Friday

Breakfast

Special K or Special K Plus
Skim or low fat milk
Fresh or unsweetened
canned fruit

Lunch

Sourdough rye with lean
roast beef and mayonnaise
or smoked salmon and
light cream cheese
Fresh fruit

Dinner

Mediterranean lasagna*
Green salad
Peaches and low fat
ice cream

Saturday

Breakfast

Sourdough French toast with
maple syrup and sliced
strawberries
Tomato juice

Lunch

Pita pizza and three-bean
salad
Fresh or unsweetened
canned fruit cocktail

Dinner

Butter bean, pepper and
shrimp pilaf*
Diced nectarine and plums
topped with low fat yogurt
and a sprinkle of toasted
almonds

Sunday

Breakfast

Western omelet
Rye toast with tub margarine
Fruit compote or crisp

Lunch

Grilled vegetables and
beans with pasta*
Large mixed green salad
with olive oil vinaigrette
Fresh fruit

Dinner

Lean lamb roast brushed
with oil, rosemary and
dried mint
Baked sweet potato fries
Fresh steamed greens
Individual apple and ginger
crumble*

7-day Glucose Revolution
Life Plan Menus

—For Biggerbodies

(an asterisk* next to a meal indicates that the recipe is included in this book.)

Monday

Breakfast
Wholegrain toast with
   peanut butter and
   apple butter
Grapefruit or tomato juice

Lunch
Hearty winter vegetable
   soup*
Small wholegrain roll
Small apple

Dinner
Cod with sun-dried tomato
   marinade*
Brown rice
Green beans
Mesclun and cherry tomato
   salad

Tuesday

Breakfast
Low fat granola
Low fat or light yogurt
Fresh strawberries

Lunch
Mixed salad (mesclun lettuce,
   cherry tomatoes, cucumber,
   celery, string beans,
   marinated mushrooms) with
   tomato-olive vinaigrette*
Cornmeal, pepper and
   chive muffin*

Dinner
Grilled chicken breast
Sweet potato, potato and
   garlic mash*, or
   corn on the cob, spinach
   and snow peas

Wednesday

Breakfast
Old-fashioned rolled oats
Dried fruit
Skim or low fat milk
Fresh grapefruit

Lunch
Turkey, lettuce and
   tomato sandwich on
Sliced cantaloupe

Dinner
Vegetable sesame noodle
   stir-fry*
Softly simmered
   peaches* topped with
   a dollop of light
   vanilla yogurt

Thursday

Breakfast

Multigrain toast with a
smear of canola margarine
Boiled egg
Tomato juice

Lunch

Toasted pita bread with
hummus* and tabouli
Fruit smoothie

Dinner

Pork fillet with spiced pears
and basmati rice*
Steamed carrot and zucchini
or other fresh vegetables

Friday

Breakfast

Special K or Special K Plus
Skim or low fat milk
Small piece of fruit
Skim milk cappuccino

Lunch

A sandwich made with
low G.I. bread with salmon,
lettuce and tomato
Fresh fruit

Dinner

Mediterranean lasagna*
Green salad
Peaches and a scoop of
low fat ice cream

Saturday

Breakfast

Sourdough French toast
Canadian bacon
Maple syrup
Sliced strawberries
Tomato juice

Lunch

Vegetable pasta salad
(small pasta shells, tuna,
chopped tomato, celery,
cucumber and parsley);
dress with balsamic
vinaigrette or a tablespoon
of light mayonnaise

Dinner

Butter bean, pepper and
shrimp pilaf*
Diced nectarine and plums
with a dollop of low fat
vanilla yogurt
Slice of zucchini or
pumpkin bread

Sunday

Breakfast

Western omelet
Rye toast with tub margarine
Fruit compote

Lunch

Grilled tomato and
eggplant and part skim
mozzarella
Large mixed green salad
with olive oil vinaigrette

Dinner

Lean lamb roast brushed
with oil, rosemary and
dried mint
Grilled garlic potatoes
and sweet potato*
Fresh steamed greens
Fresh fruit plate

7-day Glucose Revolution Life Plan Menus

—For Kidsbodies

(an asterisk* next to a meal indicates that the recipe is included in this book.)

Monday

Breakfast
Strawberry-banana smoothie
   with vanilla yogurt
   and honey

Snack
Graham crackers

Lunch
Ham sandwich with
   lettuce and tomatoes
Small apple and
   mini yogurt

Snack
Orange quarters

Dinner
Barbecued chicken with
   corn on the cob and salad
Pear halves

Tuesday

Breakfast
Apricot and muesli muffin*
   Bowl of fruit salad with
   low fat or light yogurt

Snack
Low fat granola bar

Lunch
Turkey and tomato
   sandwich on low G.I.
   bread, spread with
   light mayonnaise

Snack
Sliced fresh fruit

Dinner
Oven fried fish sticks (Choose
   products cooked in canola
   oil)
Steamed broccoli
Peaches

Wednesday

Breakfast
Low G.I. toast with peanut
   butter and all-fruit jelly

Snack
Low fat or light yogurt

Lunch
Melted cheese sandwich
   made with low
   G.I. bread

Snack
Grapes

Dinner
Chunky chicken-vegetable
   noodle soup
Whole grain roll spread with
   tub margarine
Baked apple

Thursday

Breakfast
Special K with skim or
  low fat milk
Strawberries or peaches

Snack
Snack pack of natural
  applesauce

Lunch
Tuna salad sandwich,
  made with low G.I.
  bread
Grapes

Snack
Sliced fresh fruit

Dinner
Hamburger on 100% whole
  wheat bun
Baked beans
Large tossed salad
Low fat chocolate milk

Friday

Breakfast
Scrambled eggs
Whole grain toast spread
  with tub margarine
Grapes

Snack
A slice of cheese and
  whole wheat crackers

Lunch
Peanut butter and all fruit
  jelly on low G.I. bread
Snack pack of peaches
Grapes

Snack
Fruit yogurt
Chocolate chip cookies

Dinner
Mediterranean lasagna*
Tossed salad
Fresh strawberries with a
  scoop of low fat ice cream

Saturday

Breakfast
Sourdough French toast
  with maple syrup
Sliced fruit

Snack
Mini oat bites*
Glass of skim or low fat milk

Lunch
Pita pizza
Tossed green salad
Skim or lowfat milk

Snack
Baby carrots
Chocolate chip cookies

Dinner
Vegetable sesame noodle
  stir fry*
Low fat ice cream with sliced
  banana, nuts and 1 tbsp.
  chocolate syrup

Sunday

Breakfast
Buckwheat pancakes with
  maple syrup and
  sliced fruit

Snack
Piece of fresh fruit

Lunch
Spaghetti with
  Mediterranean pasta
  sauce and cheese
A bowl of small chunks
  of fresh fruit offered
  with toothpicks and
  yogurt to dip

Snack
Cheese and fruit plate
  with water crackers

Dinner
Lean roast beef with mashed
  sweet potato and green beans
Apple crisp

7-day Glucose Revolution Life Plan Menus

—For Busybodies

(an asterisk* next to a meal indicates that the recipe is included in this book.)

We have indicated the G.I. rating of the carbohydrate foods in the following meals and snacks to help you choose the right type of food for your circumstances.

Monday

Breakfast

Wholegrain fruit and nut loaf, toasted and topped with light cream cheese, slices of apple, and cinnamon
A glass of low fat milk

Lunch

Tuna salad sandwiches on mixed grain bread
A large pear

Dinner

Garlic prawns, pepper and cilantro pasta
Green salad
Bread roll
Fresh low G.I. fruit

Tuesday

Breakfast

Large serving of chunky fresh fruit salad topped with light yogurt and low fat granola
Apricot and muesli muffin

Lunch

Large bowl of split pea soup
Tomato and cucumber salad
Apple
Skim or low fat flavored milk

Dinner

Roasted sweet potato, garlic and rosemary pilaf
Summer pudding

Wednesday

Breakfast

Old fashioned rolled oats cooked with mixed dried fruit topped with pecans or walnuts
Toast with honey
Skim or low fat milk

Lunch

Roast beef and turkey club sandwich on low G.I. bread
Tomato or V-8 juice

Dinner

Antipasto (vegetarian) with bread
Vegetarian pizza
Gelato

Thursday

Breakfast

Multigrain waffles with
applesauce
Skim milk cappuccino

Lunch

Hamburger on a toasted
bun served with lettuce,
sliced tomato and chili
sauce
Baked sweet potato fries
Flavored mineral water

Dinner

Rack of lamb with lemon
and rosemary on
potato-garlic mash
Bread roll
Poached pears with
low fat, no sugar added
vanilla yogurt and
toasted sliced almonds

Friday

Breakfast

Baked ham and melted light
cheese on whole grain
bread
Canned peach slices

Lunch

Smoked salmon and light
cream cheese on
pumpernickel bread
Carrot salad
Fruit salad

Dinner

Meatloaf with a whole grain
roll
Fresh cantaloupe with
low fat ice cream

Saturday

Breakfast

100% stoneground whole
nwheat toast with peanut
butter and all-fruit jelly
Orange

Lunch

Marinated BBQ chicken
noodle salad
Canned fruit

Dinner

Tenderloin pork medallions
with mushroom gravy and
pureed cauliflower
Baked cinnamon apple

Sunday

Breakfast

All Bran with Extra Fiber
with light yogurt and
berries
A couple of slices of
wholegrain toast with
all-fruit jelly
An apple

Lunch

Spaghetti with basic tomato
sauce and cheese
Semolina garlic bread
Fresh fruit salad

Dinner

Seared tuna with
red pepper coulis
Creamed corn
Creamed corn
Fresh fruit platter

Snacks

Trail mix
Raisin toast
Fresh fruit
Skim or low fat milk with
chocolate flavoring
Low fat yogurt
A fruit smoothie

Muffins (see our recipes)
Snack packs of canned fruit
Crackers and jelly
Peanuts
Graham crackers
Baked tortilla chips
and salsa

Oatmeal cookies
Fig bars
Dried apricots
Low fat granola bars
Toast and honey
Bowl of NutriGrain™
or Special K

The Glucose Revolution Life Plan Shopper:
Keeping a Well-Stocked Kitchen

IN THE PANTRY

Dried herbs and spices
   Whole black peppercorns
   Chili powder
   Ground cumin and coriander
   Prepared mustard, e.g. Dijon and whole seed

Oils and vinegars
   Extra virgin olive oil
   Canola oil
   Sunola™
   Sesame oil
   White wine vinegar
   Red wine vinegar
   Balsamic vinegar

Grain foods
   Pasta and noodles (fresh and dried)
   Brown rice, Basmati rice, Uncle Ben's converted rice
   Couscous
   Polenta (cornmeal)
   Pearl barley
   Cracked wheat (bulgur)

Legumes
   Canned of all types
   Dried lentils and split peas

Sauces
   Soy sauce
   Oyster sauce
   Fish sauce
   Chinese rice wine
   Chili sauce
   Bottled tomato pasta sauce (such as marinara)
   Curry pastes

The Glucose Revolution Life Plan Shopper: Keeping a Well-Stocked Kitchen

Bottled foods
Sundried tomatoes
Artichoke hearts
Olives
Capers
Marinated feta cheese
Marinated vegetables
Roasted red peppers
Pickles

Canned food
Tuna packed in spring water or oil
Salmon packed in water
Sardines packed in water, oil or tomato sauce
Tomatoes and tomato paste
Corn
Fruits

Note: Fish canned in oil contains about 10 times more fat than fish canned in water. If you prefer to buy tuna in oil, check the ingredient list closely for the type of oil used: Canola, olive or soybean is best.

Nuts, seeds and dried fruit
Almonds, walnuts, pine nuts, pecans, apricots
Sesame seeds, sunflower seeds, flaxseeds

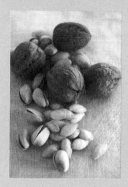

The Glucose Revolution Life Plan Shopper: Keeping a Well-Stocked Kitchen

IN THE FRIDGE

Low fat or skim milk
Canola margarine
Canola mayonnaise
Parmesan cheese
Light ricotta cheese
Reduced fat cheddar
Light or low fat plain and fruit yogurt
Fresh pasta and noodles
Fresh vegetables, including green leafy vegetables: lettuce, spinach, eggplant, cabbage, broccoli, cauliflower
Lemons
Onions
Tomatoes
Fresh herbs such as parsley and basil
Ginger, garlic, chili: bottled or fresh

Note: If you buy fresh ginger and need to keep it more than a week, peel it, place in a jar, cover with oil and refrigerate; or peel, place in a freezer bag and freeze.

IN THE FREEZER

Peas, beans
Frozen spinach
Mixed vegetables
Reduced fat ice cream or sorbet
Frozen berries

Part Three

50

glucose
life plan
RECIPES

CHAPTER 10

About the Recipes

NOW THAT YOU can distinguish between low and high G.I. foods, how about some recipes to put your knowledge into practice and turn mealtimes into healthy and delicious events? The recipes we've chosen aren't gourmet—they're just delicious, low G.I. and super easy to make. (We know that you probably don't have a lot of time to cook!) And they're full of healthy ingredients such as fish and seafood, legumes, whole grains, olive oil and fresh fruit and vegetables.

Our recipes are based on a dietary philosophy that emphasizes:

- low G.I. carbohydrate, with carbohydrate meeting 40 to 50 percent of calorie requirements;
- monounsaturated fats and omega-3 fats, with 30 to 35 percent of calories coming from fat; and
- a moderate level of protein providing 15 to 20 percent of calories.

nutrition information

We've included nutrition information with each recipe, including calories, protein, fat, carbohydrate and fiber content per serving. Where there is a range in the number of servings the recipe yields, the nutrition information relates to the larger number of servings.

energy requirements

In keeping with our dietary philosophy, we recommend the following levels of macronutrients for various energy requirements. (These energy levels are an approximate guide only, and assume good health status and a moderate level of activity.)

An average energy requirement for young to middle-aged men:
    2400 calories, made up of 90 to 120 grams protein,
    80 to 95 grams fat, 250 to 300 grams carbohydrate.

An average energy requirement for young to middle-aged women and older men, and a reduced energy intake for younger men:
    2000 calories made up of 75 to 100 grams protein,
    70 to 80 grams fat, 210 to 250 grams carbohydrate.

An average energy requirement for older women, a reduced energy intake for young to middle-aged women, and a low energy intake for men:
    1500 calories made up of 55 to 75 grams protein,
    50 to 60 grams fat, 150 to 200 grams carbohydrate.

A low energy intake for young to middle-aged women:
    1200 calories made up of 45 to 60 grams protein,
    40 to 45 grams fat, 125 to 150 grams carbohydrate.

fat

We've minimized saturated fat and increased unsaturated fat. We've made a particular effort to increase omega-3 fats in the recipes and use omega-neutral monounsaturates. We've estimated the amount of omega-3 fats for each recipe and have indicated the amount with a star rating that reflects the quantity per serving.

Those of you who have been following a low fat diet may be surprised by the fat content of some of the recipes. Dietary guidelines are changing: There is a move away from very low fat diets as science reveals the health benefits of certain types of fats. It is important, however, to remember that an increase in fat intake will result in an increase in calorie intake unless you also reduce the amount of another nutrient, such as carbohydrate.

Because of this, we feel that a higher fat diet will not suit everyone. In particular, those people who have a big appetite and like to eat a large volume of food could control their weight more easily on a low fat–high carbohydrate diet. Low fat, high carbohydrate foods are less energy dense than higher fat foods, which means that it is possible to eat a larger volume of them while still eating within caloric requirements.

If you are trying to lose weight, and sometimes struggle with hunger, try to stick to the lower fat intakes for the various energy levels recommended above. For example, for a young to middle-aged woman on a reduced calorie intake of about 1500 calories, aiming for around 50 grams of fat per day allows a more generous amount of carbohydrate in the diet at 200 grams per day.

omega-3 rating

>1000 milligrams per serving	*****	One of the richest sources of omega-3s
500-1000 milligrams per serving	****	A very good source of omega-3s
100-500 milligrams per serving	***	A good source of omega-3s
50-100 milligrams per serving	**	Valuable amounts of omega-3s
<50 milligrams per serving	*	A small amount of omega-3s

If you don't see an omega-3 rating, it means that there's negligible omega-3 content in that recipe. Saturated fat provides less than 10 percent of the energy content of all recipes except where specifically stated otherwise in the nutrient information.

carbohydrate

Many of the recipes are carbohydrate-based, but we emphasize low G.I. carbohydrate. Each recipe has a G.I. ranking according to whether its G.I. value is low, moderate or high. The following table gives approximate G.I. values for these different rankings.

Low carbohydrate recipes have little effect on our blood glucose levels, so we have given them a G.I. rating of zero.

g.i. rating

Low G.I. = a G.I. value of less than 55
Moderate G.I. = a G.I. value of 56–69
High G.I. = a G.I. value greater than 70

protein

There is evidence that we evolved on much higher protein intakes than we eat today, although there's insufficient evidence yet to suggest that we need to greatly increase our protein intake. Protein foods are a critical source of some nutrients such as iron (from red meat) and omega-3 fats (from fish and seafood). Most people consume 15 to 20 percent of energy as protein, which is in line with current guidelines. The protein content of these recipes varies according to the main ingredients; the entrees based on meat, fish or legumes are higher in protein than recipes based entirely on vegetables.

fiber

A diet rich in fruits and vegetables will be naturally high in fiber. The typical American diet contains about 20 grams of fiber a day, which falls far short of the recommendation that we should eat 30 to 40 grams every day. The daily fiber requirements of children and adolescents are estimated as their age in years plus five: This gives the number of grams of fiber recommended per day.

Most of the recipes in this book are high in fiber, providing an average of 5 grams of fiber per serving.

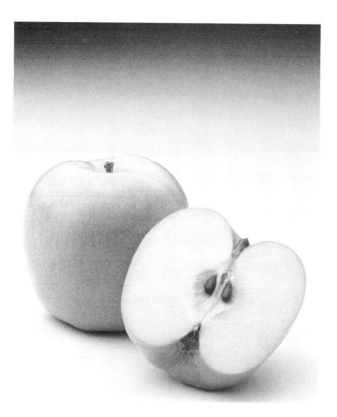

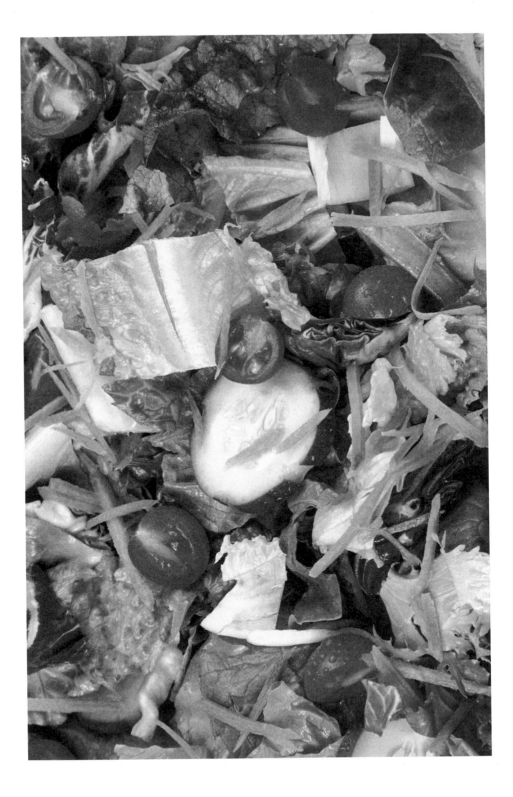

CHAPTER 11

Snacks, Soups, Salads and Sauces

Baby Spinach Salad

 low

CALORIES: 159
PROTEIN: 7G
FAT: 13G
CARBOHYDRATE: 5G
FIBER: 1G
OMEGA-3: *

4 cups baby spinach

small shallot, thinly sliced

½ pint (4 ozs.) grape tomatoes, halved

2 hard boiled eggs, horizontally sliced

1 tablespoon Parmesan cheese, grated

2 strips bacon, crisply cooked and diced

¼ cup vinaigrette dressing

1. Wash and pat spinach leaves dry. Trim off long stalks.
2. Layer first four ingredients in large salad plate.
3. Sprinkle top layer with cheese and bacon.
4. Drizzle with dressing.
5. Toss and serve.

Serves 4 • Preparation time: 20 minutes

Stir-Fried Greens

 G low

CALORIES: 29
PROTEIN: 2G
FAT: 2G
CARBOHYDRATE: 2G
FIBER: 1G
OMEGA-3: **

1 ½ lbs. leafy greens (such as bok choy,
Swiss chard, kale, Savoy cabbage)
1 tablespoon oil, sesame or peanut
½ tablespoon fresh garlic, minced
½ tablespoon fresh ginger, minced
1 tablespoon soy sauce

1. Separate leaves and trim stalks. Rinse and pat dry.
2. Chop coarsely.
3. Heat oil in a wok.
4. Add greens, stir-fry 2 minutes.
5. Add garlic and ginger, then continue stir-frying for another
   1–2 minutes.
6. Sprinkle soy sauce and stir thoroughly. Serve immediately.

Makes 4 cups

Serves 8 • Preparation time: 15 minutes • Cooking time: 5 minutes

Spinach with Honey-Soy Dressing

Ⓖ low

CALORIES: 42
PROTEIN: 3G
FAT: 1G
CARBOHYDRATE: 7G
FIBER: 3G
OMEGA-3: *

20 ozs. fresh spinach
1 tablespoon honey, warmed
1 tablespoon soy sauce
1 teaspoon sesame oil
1 teaspoon sesame seeds, toasted

1. Wash, drain and trim spinach leaves.
2. With just the water that adheres to the leaves, cover spinach and microwave on HIGH for 2 minutes.
3. Remove from microwave and carefully squeeze out all excess liquid. (Spinach will be very hot!)
4. In a screw-top jar combine next four ingredients (honey through sesame seeds). Shake well.
5. Pour dressing over cooked spinach and toss well. Serve immediately.

Makes 3 cups

Serves 6 • Preparation time: 10 minutes • Cooking time: 2 minutes

Roasted Sweet Potato

 low

CALORIES: 143
PROTEIN: 2G
FAT: 2G
CARBOHYDRATE: 29G
FIBER: 2G

2 lbs. sweet potatoes

1 tablespoon olive oil

½ tablespoon fresh or dried rosemary

⅛ teaspoon black pepper

1. Preheat oven to 375°F.
2. Peel the potatoes and cut into 1-inch cubes.
3. Microwave on high for 6 minutes, until the outside begins to soften.
4. Drain the potatoes and transfer them to a baking pan sprayed with cooking spray.
5. Brush potatoes with the olive oil and sprinkle with rosemary and pepper.
6. Bake in oven approximately 25 minutes or until tender. Serve immediately.

Serves 6–8 • Preparation time: 5 minutes • Cooking time: 30 minutes

Meatless Mediterranean Roast

 low

CALORIES: 155
PROTEIN: 3G
FAT: 5G
CARBOHYDRATE: 27G
FIBER: 5G

1 lb. sweet potatoes (3 medium-sized)

1 lb. zucchini (3 medium-sized)

1 large red onion

2 red peppers

2 tablespoons olive oil

salt and pepper to taste

3 sprigs fresh rosemary

3 garlic cloves, halved

1. Preheat oven to 400°F.
2. Peel sweet potatoes. Wash and pat dry and cut into 1½-inch chunks. Place in large mixing bowl. Wash, pat dry and cut zucchini into 1-inch thick round slices. Add to the mixing bowl.
4. Peel and cut onion into 8 wedges; add to mixing bowl.
5. Wash and seed peppers and cut each one lengthwise into 12 slices.
6. Pour olive oil over vegetables. Add salt, pepper, rosemary and garlic. Toss well to coat thoroughly.
7. Place vegetables in 13 x 9 x 2¼ baking pan.
8. Bake in preheated oven for 40 minutes.

Makes 6 cups

Serves 6 • Preparation time: 20 minutes • Cooking time: 40 minutes

Slow-Roasted Tomatoes

 low

CALORIES: 61
PROTEIN: 2G
FAT: 3G
CARBOHYDRATE: 7G
FIBER: 2G

2 lbs. fresh, ripe tomatoes

1 tablespoon olive oil

1 tablespoon balsamic vinegar

pepper to taste

½ tablespoon crushed garlic
or ½ teaspoon garlic powder

1 tablespoon pesto

1. Preheat oven to 350°F.
2. Bring 2 quarts water to a boil.
3. Wash the tomatoes and place in a deep bowl; cover them with the boiling water. Let stand 2 minutes.
4. Drain and peel off skins.
5. Cut the tomatoes in half and place cut-side up in a large, shallow baking pan.
6. Combine the oil, vinegar, pepper, garlic and pesto and brush on tomato halves.
7. Bake for 25 minutes.

Serves 6 • Preparation time: 5 minutes • Cooking time: 25 minutes

Softly Simmered Peaches

 low

CALORIES: 49
PROTEIN: 1G
FAT: 0G
CARBOHYDRATE: 10G
FIBER: 2G

4 ripe peaches, halved and pitted
1 teaspoon sugar
dash ground cinnamon
pinch ground nutmeg (optional)

1. Blanch pear halves for easy peeling: Drop fruit in boiling water for 2 minutes; run under cold water; peel back skin with knife.
2. Place peach halves, cut side down, in 9-inch-square pan with 1 inch of boiling water, sprinkle with sugar and spices.
3. Cover and simmer until tender, about 10 minutes. Serve warm or at room temperature.

Serves 4 • Preparation time: 5 minutes • Cooking time: 5 minutes

Poached Pears

G low

CALORIES: 200
PROTEIN: 1G
FAT: 1G
CARBOHYDRATE: 51G
FIBER: 3G

4 Bosc pears, just ripe

water

½ cup sugar

1 cinnamon stick

1 teaspoon vanilla extract

1 tablespoon brandy

1. Cut pears in half. Peel and core; set aside.
2. In medium saucepan mix water, sugar and cinnamon stick. Bring to a boil, then simmer uncovered for 10 minutes, or until a thin syrup forms.
3. Add vanilla and brandy to syrup. Swirl to mix.
4. Place pear halves, cut-side down, in saucepan. Bring to boil, then cover and let simmer for about 15 minutes or until tender.
5. Serve warm with a thin vanilla or chocolate sauce or plain at room temperature.

Serves 4 • Preparation time: 10 minutes • Cooking time: 25 minutes

Chick Nuts

 low

CALORIES: 157
PROTEIN: 5G
FAT: 6G
CARBOHYDRATE: 22G
FIBER: 5G
OMEGA-3: **

Spice mixture:

½ teaspoon each: cumin, chili powder, paprika, ground coriander, salt

2 teaspoons sugar

19 oz.-can chickpeas, drained

1 tablespoon oil (peanut or canola)

1. Prepare spice mixture in small bowl.
2. Place chickpeas in large mixing bowl. Sprinkle spice mixture over chickpeas. Toss well to thoroughly coat.
3. Heat oil in large frying pan. Add chickpeas and cook for 5 minutes, stirring frequently so "nuts" brown evenly.
4. Transfer chickpeas onto paper towel to cool thoroughly.
5. Store in airtight container for up to one week.

Makes 2 cups

Serves 4 • Preparation time: 10 minutes • Cooking time: 5 minutes

Pepper, Corn and Barley Patties

 low

CALORIES: 115
PROTEIN: 3G
FAT: 4G
CARBOHYDRATE: 16G
FIBER: 3G
OMEGA-3: **

1 lb. sweet potato, peeled

1 cup quick-cook barley
(from health food stores)

1 15¼ oz. can corn kernels, drained

1 medium red pepper, halved,
seeded and diced small

½ bunch flat leafed or curly parsley,
finely chopped (approx. ½ cup)

1 egg, lightly beaten

salt and freshly ground black pepper

2 tablespoons canola oil

1. Cut the sweet potato into chunks and boil in plenty of water until soft. Drain, mash until smooth, and place in a large mixing bowl.

2. Add the raw barley, drained corn kernels, diced pepper and chopped parsley. Blend in the beaten egg with a large spoon, and season with salt and freshly ground pepper.

3. Heat the oil in a heavy frying pan. Shape the patties with wet hands, and cook for 5 minutes, turning once only, until golden brown.

Makes 8 large or 12 small patties

Preparation time: 10 minutes • Cooking time: 20 minutes

Cornmeal, Pepper and Chive Muffins

(G) **moderate**

CALORIES: 208
PROTEIN: 6G
FAT: 7G
CARBOHYDRATE: 31G
FIBER: 2G
OMEGA-3: **

3 tablespoons canola oil

2 tablespoons honey

1 1/2 cups buttermilk

1 egg

1 15 1/4 oz. can corn kernels, drained

1 medium red pepper, finely diced

1 bunch chives, snipped

1 cup cornmeal/polenta

1 1/2 cups self-raising flour

pinch salt

1. Preheat the oven to 375°F.
2. Lightly oil or spray a 12-muffin tray.
3. In a large mixing bowl, beat together the oil, honey, buttermilk and egg. Add the corn kernels, diced pepper and chives, then quickly stir in the cornmeal, flour and salt.
4. Spoon the muffin mixture into the prepared tin, and bake for 25 to 30 minutes, until cooked through and golden brown.

Makes 12

Preparation time: 20 minutes • Cooking time: 30 minutes

Apricot and Muesli Muffins

Ⓖ moderate

CALORIES: 237
PROTEIN: 5G
FAT: 7G
CARBOHYDRATE: 38G
FIBER: 4G
OMEGA-3: **

1 cup (about 6 oz.) plump dried apricots, coarsely chopped

1 1/2 cups unsweetened natural muesli

2 cups (8 oz.) self-raising flour

1 teaspoon baking powder

1 cup apple juice

3 tablespoons canola oil

1/4 cup honey

1 egg

1. Preheat the oven to 375°F.
2. Lightly oil or spray a 12-muffin tray.
3. In a large mixing bowl mix together the chopped apricots, muesli, self-raising flour and baking powder.
4. In another bowl combine the apple juice, oil, honey and egg. Add the flour mixture to the liquid mix and stir until just combined.
5. Spoon the muffin mixture into the prepared muffin tins and bake for 20 minutes, until brown and cooked through.

Makes 12

Preparation time: 10 minutes • Cooking time: 20 minutes

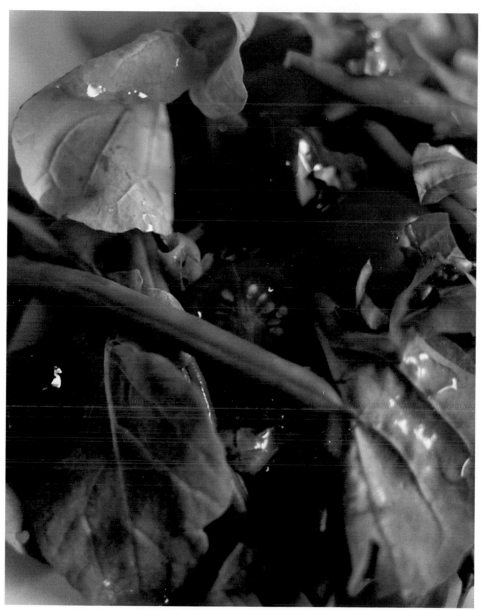

Green Bean, Arugula, Cherry Tomato and Olive Salad

▶ page 162

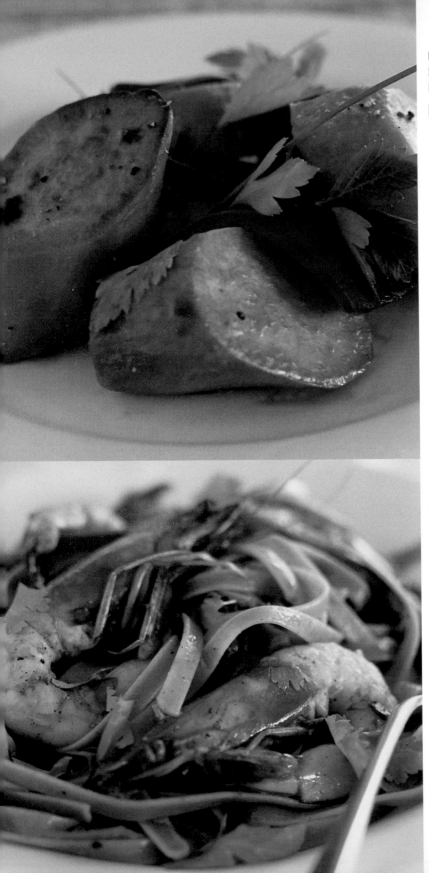

Grilled Pepper, Sweet Potato and Herb Salad

▶ page 163

Garlic Prawns, Pepper and Cilantro Pasta

▶ page 172

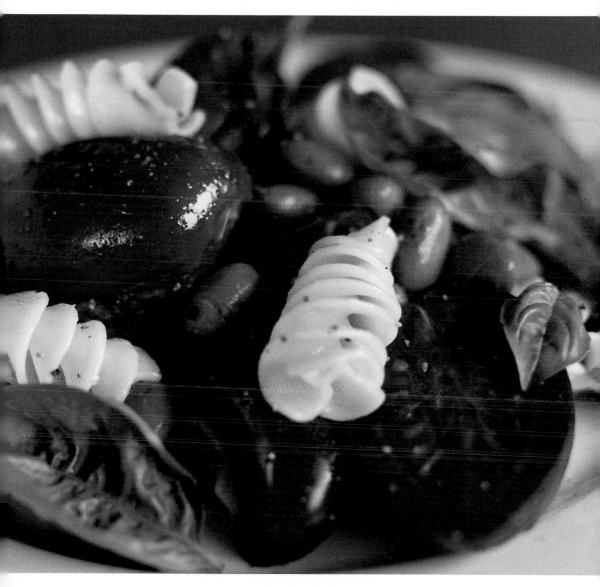

Grilled Vegetables and Beans with Pasta ▶ page 170

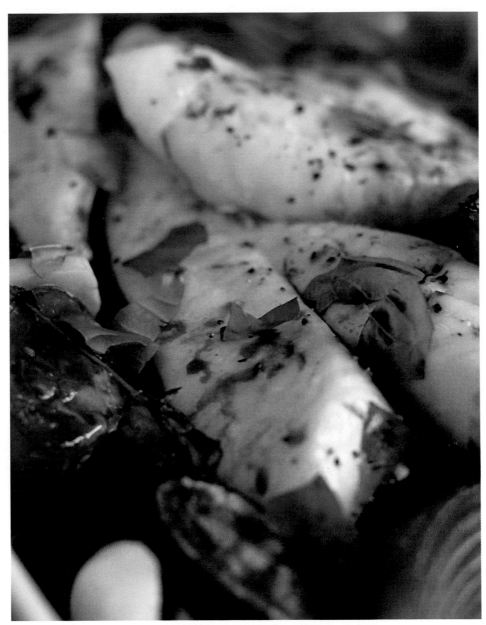

Deep Sea Perch on Roasted Vegetables ▶ page 197

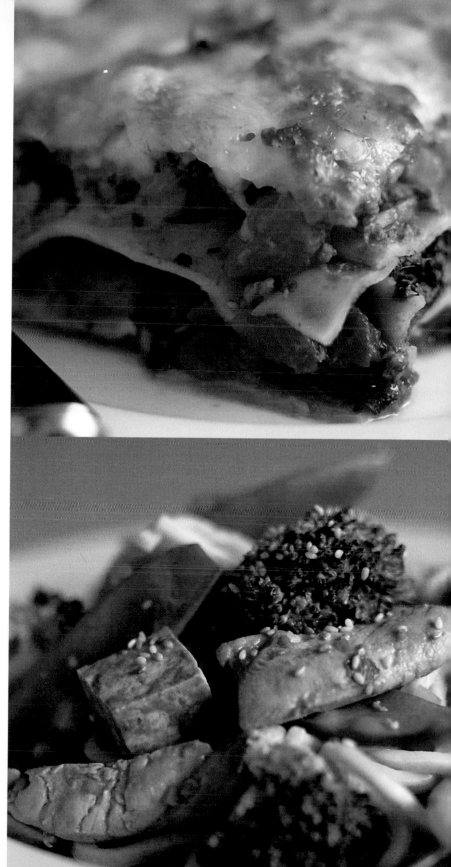

Mediterranean Lasagna

▶ page 201

Tofu Chicken with Snow Peas and Rice Noodles

▶ page 175

**Cornmeal,
Pepper and
Chive Muffins**

▶ page 149

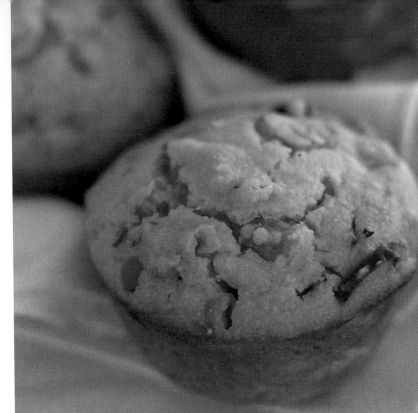

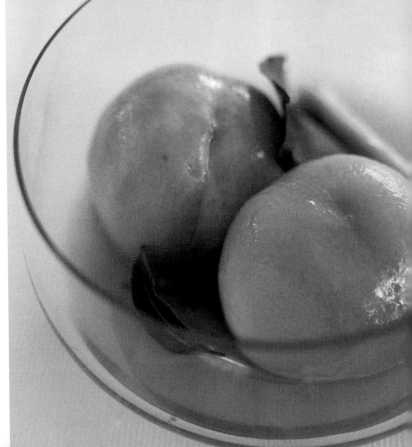

**Poached
Peaches in
Lemon-Ginger
Syrup**

▶ page 209

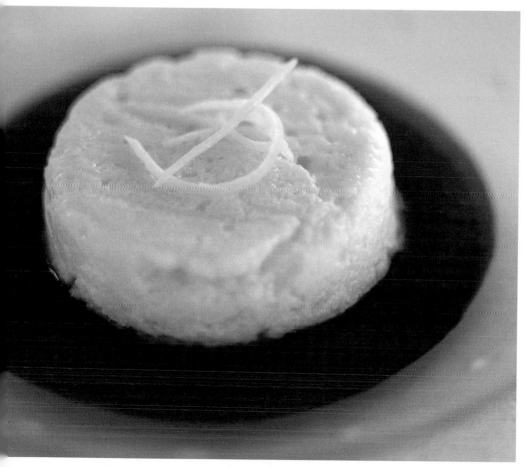

Lemon Semolina Pudding with Berry Coulis ▶ page 211

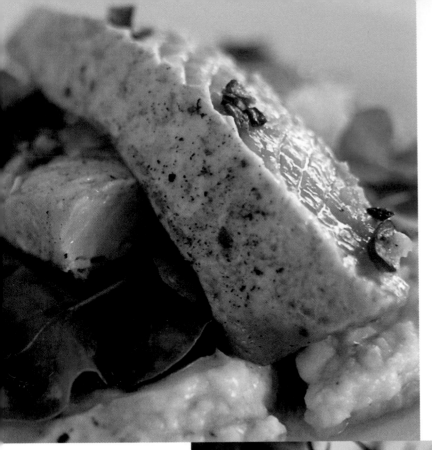

**Seared Atlantic
Salmon Fillets with
White Bean Puree**

▶ page 202

**Rack of Lamb
with Lemon
and Rosemary
on Potato-
Garlic
Mash**

▶ page 193

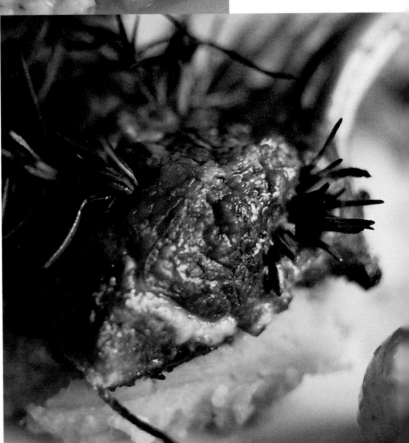

Chocolate Chip Muffins

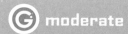 **moderate**

CALORIES: 280
PROTEIN: 7G
FAT: 8G
CARBOHYDRATE: 46G
FIBER: 2G
OMEGA-3: **

1 cup sifted whole wheat flour
1 cup sifted all-purpose flour
1 tablespoon baking powder
1 cup dark brown sugar, lightly packed
1 tablespoon mixed spice
1 cup chocolate chips
1 cup buttermilk
1 teaspoon vanilla extract
2 eggs
1 tablespoon canola oil

1. Preheat the oven to 375°F and lightly oil or spray a 12-muffin tray.
2. In one bowl mix together the flours, baking powder, sugar and mixed spice. Fold in the chocolate chips.
3. In another large mixing bowl whisk together the buttermilk, vanilla extract, eggs and canola oil.
4. Quickly stir the dry ingredients into the buttermilk mixture and spoon into the prepared muffin tray.
5. Place in the preheated oven and bake for 25 minutes, until brown and cooked through.

Makes 12

Preparation time: 10 minutes • Cooking time: 25 minutes

G low

CALORIES: 139
PROTEIN: 6G
FAT: 10G
CARBOHYDRATE: 5G
FIBER: 4G
OMEGA-3: *

1 15-oz. can chickpeas
½ cup tahini (sesame seed paste)
2 cloves garlic, coarsely chopped
⅓ cup lemon juice
salt and freshly ground black pepper

1. Drain the chickpeas and reserve the liquid.
2. In a food processor, combine the chickpeas, tahini paste, garlic, lemon juice and seasonings. Process, adding enough reserved chickpea liquid to make a smooth consistency.
3. Serve with a low G.I. bread as a dip, in place of butter in sandwiches, or layered with grilled vegetables on focaccia.

Makes 2 cups

NOTE: Nutrition information below is for one ¼ cup-serving

Preparation time: 15 minutes

Baby Pea and Ham Soup

 low

CALORIES: 121
PROTEIN: 12G
FAT: 1G
CARBOHYDRATE: 15G
FIBER: 10G

1 large smoked ham bone

2 quarts water

1 ½ lbs. carrots (about 4 large), diced

4 celery stalks, diced

3 large onions, finely diced

3 bay leaves

1 lb. (approx.) frozen baby peas

½ bunch parsley, coarsely chopped

freshly ground black pepper

1. Place the ham bone and water in a large saucepan and bring to a boil. Remove any froth that forms on the surface. Simmer for 5 minutes, then add the prepared carrots, celery, onions and bay leaves.

2. Simmer gently for 40 minutes, removing any scum as it appears. Remove the bone from the water, cut off any meat and dice. Discard the fat and skin.

3. Return the diced ham to the saucepan and add the peas, simmering gently until tender.

4. Add the chopped parsley, season with pepper and serve hot with thick slices of low G.I. toast.

Serves 6 • Preparation time: 10 minutes • Cooking time: 50 minutes

Sweet Potato, Carrot and Ginger Soup

 low

CALORIES: 183
PROTEIN: 5G
FAT: 5G
CARBOHYDRATE: 27G
FIBER: 9G

2 lbs. sweet potato, peeled and
cut into large pieces

2 lbs. carrots, peeled and
cut into large pieces

1 large onion, peeled and quartered

2 cloves garlic, peeled and coarsely chopped

4 cups chicken or vegetable stock

1½ teaspoons lemon zest

1½ teaspoons lemon juice

6 ozs. evaporated fat-free milk

⅔ cup water

Small piece fresh ginger (½" x 1"),
peeled and finely chopped

salt and freshly ground black pepper

cilantro leaves

1. Place the prepared sweet potato, carrots, onion and garlic into a large
   saucepan or stockpot.
2. Add the chicken stock and lemon zest pieces and simmer until the vegetables are soft. Remove the lemon zest pieces, add the evaporated milk,
   lemon juice, water and chopped ginger, and cook for a further 5 minutes.
3. Puree the soup until smooth, season to taste with salt and pepper and garnish with cilantro leaves. Serve hot with slices of oat bran bread.

Serves 6 • Preparation time: 10 minutes • Cooking time: 25 minutes

Hearty Winter Vegetable Soup

 low

CALORIES: 103
PROTEIN: 8G
FAT: 3G
CARBOHYDRATE: 11G
FIBER: 5G
OMEGA-3: •

8 ozs. dried lentils

4 cups chicken or vegetable stock

1 large leek, washed and finely sliced

6 stalks celery, finely sliced

1 large can (28 oz.) whole peeled tomatoes, undrained

1⅔ cups canned tomato puree

pinch of salt and freshly ground black pepper

½ bunch flat leafed parsley, coarsely chopped

2 ozs. Parmesan cheese, shaved from the block

1. Combine the lentils and the stock. Bring to a boil, cover and simmer for 45 minutes.
2. Stir in the next 6 ingredients (leek through pepper). Simmer for 15 minutes.
3. Stir in the coarsely chopped parsley and ladle into soup bowls.
3. Sprinkle each bowl with the shaved Parmesan and serve with thick slices of low G.I. toasted bread.

Serves 8 • Preparation time: 5 minutes • Cooking time: 1 hour

Roast Chicken, Garlic and Bean Soup

 low

CALORIES: 306
PROTEIN: 43G
FAT: 12G
CARBOHYDRATE: 8G
FIBER: 5G
OMEGA-3: **

6 whole cloves garlic

1 3-lb. roasted chicken (no stuffing)

2 quarts low salt chicken stock or consommé

1 tablespoon fresh thyme or 1 teaspoon dried

zest of one lemon

2 small celery stalks, finely sliced

1 15.5-oz. can light red kidney
(borlotti) beans, drained

salt and freshly ground black pepper

half bunch flat leafed parsley, coarsely chopped

1. Preheat the oven to 350°F.
2. Prick each unpeeled clove of garlic with a sharp knife and place on a baking tray. Bake in preheated oven for 20 minutes. Remove, peel and mash.
3. Remove the skin from the chicken and cut the flesh (in small pieces) from the bones. Discard the carcass.
4. Pour stock into a large saucepan and add the roasted garlic mash, thyme leaves, lemon zest, celery, and beans. Season with salt and pepper. Bring stock to a boil, simmer gently for 5 minutes, then add the chicken pieces.
5. Taste for flavor and serve with coarsely chopped parsley scattered over the top.

Serves 4–6 • Preparation time: 10 minutes • Cooking time: 25 minutes

Pumpkin, Sweet Potato and Cumin Dhal Soup

 low

CALORIES: 386
PROTEIN: 27G
FAT: 5G
CARBOHYDRATE: 59G
FIBER: 17G
OMEGA-3: **

4 ½ lbs. pumpkin
2 large sweet potatoes
2 large red onions
2 cloves garlic
1 teaspoon canola oil
2 quarts chicken or vegetable stock
2 cups dried red lentils
1 tablespoon cumin
salt and freshly ground black pepper
½ bunch flat leafed parsley

1. Peel and cut the pumpkin, sweet potato and onions into pieces. Finely chop the garlic.

2. Heat the oil in a large, heavy saucepan and toss the pumpkin, sweet potato, onions and garlic for 3 minutes over a moderate heat. Add the chicken stock, lentils, and cumin, and simmer for 30 minutes or until the pumpkin is very soft.

3. Blend the contents together until smooth and season with a little salt and pepper. Reheat, garnish with coarsely chopped parsley, and serve with warm crusty bread.

Serves 4–6 • Preparation time: 10 minutes • Cooking time: 40 minutes

Chunky Vegetable, Chicken and Pasta Soup

 low

CALORIES: 347
PROTEIN: 23G
FAT: 4G
CARBOHYDRATE: 54G
FIBER: 9G
OMEGA-3: *

2 quarts chicken or vegetable stock

4 large carrots, diced

2 large sweet potatoes, diced

2 large onions, diced

6 Brussels sprouts, cut in half

3 stalks celery, diced

1 15¼-oz. can corn niblets, drained

4 ozs. uncooked spirali pasta

4 skinless chicken thighs, trimmed of all fat and sliced

4 stalks flat leafed parsley, coarsely chopped

salt and freshly ground black pepper

1. Prepare the vegetables and chicken.
2. Heat the chicken stock in a large saucepan.
3. Add the carrots, sweet potato and onions and simmer for 10 minutes. Add the corn niblets, Brussels sprouts, celery, pasta and chicken pieces and simmer gently for a further 10 minutes or until pasta is cooked.
4. Sprinkle with parsley and season to taste. Serve hot with whole grain bread.

Serves 4–6 • Preparation time: 15 minutes • Cooking time: 20 minutes

Three Bean and Basil Salad

 low

CALORIES: 166
PROTEIN: 8G
FAT: 8G
CARBOHYDRATE: 18G
FIBER: 8G
OMEGA-3: *

1 15.5-oz. can cannellini beans, drained
1 15.5-oz. can light red kidney beans, drained
1 19 oz. can red kidney beans, drained
2 cloves garlic, crushed
3 tablespoons extra virgin olive oil
1 tablespoon lemon juice
salt and freshly ground black pepper
½ bunch fresh basil leaves, torn

1. Rinse all the drained beans well under cold running water. Drain.
2. Combine the beans in a large serving bowl or flat white platter.
3. In a lidded jar, combine the garlic, olive oil, lemon juice and seasonings and shake well.
4. Pour over the beans and toss through the basil leaves.

Serves 6–8 • Preparation time: 5 minutes

Tomato, Mint and Cucumber Salad

(To accompany Mediterranean
Lasagna, page 201.)

CALORIES: 135
PROTEIN: 3G
FAT: 12G
CARBOHYDRATE: 4G
FIBER: 3G
OMEGA-3: *

1 lb. plum tomatoes (approx. 10)

2 tablespoons fresh mint, chopped

1 lb. cucumbers

15 kalamata olives

½ cup Parmesan cheese,
shaved from the block

Dressing

10 mint leaves

3 tablespoons olive oil

3 tablespoons white wine vinegar

1 clove garlic, crushed

salt and freshly ground black pepper

1. Slice the tomatoes crossways and sprinkle with chopped mint. Slice the cucumbers crossways and toss in a salad bowl with the tomatoes.
2. Add the olives and sprinkle with shaved Parmesan cheese.
3. Combine the dressing ingredients in a blender, or chop the mint and combine in a screw-top jar and shake to mix. Pour over the salad and serve immediately.

Serves 6 • Preparation time: 10 minutes

Celery, Walnut and Lemon Thyme Salad

(To accompany Fresh Fettuccine with Scallops, page 168.)

6 stalks celery

1 cup walnuts

6 sprigs lemon thyme,
leaves stripped from stalks

Dressing

1 teaspoon celery seeds

1 tablespoon lemon juice

2 tablespoons apple juice

2 tablespoons extra virgin olive oil

1 tablespoon fresh thyme leaves

salt and freshly ground black pepper

1. Wash and slice the celery sticks diagonally.
2. In a salad bowl, toss the celery with whole walnuts and thyme sprigs.
3. Place all the dressing ingredients in a screw-top jar and shake. Pour over the salad and serve with crusty low G.I. bread.

Serves 6 • Preparation time: 10 minutes

Green Bean, Arugula, Cherry Tomato and Olive Salad

(To accompany Cod Fillets with Sun-dried Tomato Marinade, page 200.)

G zero

CALORIES: 110
PROTEIN: 2G
FAT: 10G
CARBOHYDRATE: 3G
FIBER: 3G
OMEGA-3: *

$^2/_3$ lb. green beans

1 bunch arugula

1 pint cherry tomatoes

3 green shallots, finely sliced

10 kalamata olives

6 basil leaves, torn

Dressing

2 tablespoons wine vinegar

$^1/_4$ cup extra virgin olive oil

1 clove garlic, crushed

salt and freshly ground black pepper

1. Wash and trim the beans, and halve if very long. Wash the arugula, cut off stems and discard any bruised leaves. Wash the tomatoes, halve them and combine with the beans and arugula leaves on a platter or in a shallow bowl.

2. Slice the shallots, and combine in a bowl with the olives and torn basil leaves. Add to the salad vegetables.

3. Place all the dressing ingredients into a screw-top jar and shake to mix.

4. Pour the dressing over the salad.

Serves 6 • Preparation time: 15 minutes

Grilled Pepper, Sweet Potato and Herb Salad

 low

CALORIES: 166
PROTEIN: 5G
FAT: 5G
CARBOHYDRATE: 25G
FIBER: 4 G
OMEGA-3: **

2 large peppers (green, red, yellow or orange), halved and seeded

4 medium sized sweet potatoes, peeled

1 tablespoon canola or olive oil

½ bunch chives, left whole

1 bunch flat leafed parsley, coarsely chopped

salt and freshly ground black pepper

1 tablespoon balsamic vinegar

1. Preheat the grill to high. Place the pepper halves, skin side up, on the hot grill and cook until black blisters appear (about 10 minutes). Place them into a paper bag. When cool, remove the skin and cut the flesh into thick slices. (The peppers can be broiled instead of grilled if it's more convenient.)

2. Parboil the sweet potato for about 10 minutes, drain and slice diagonally. Brush each wedge with mustard seed oil. Place on a sheet of foil on the grill and cook until golden brown for approximately 15 minutes. (Sweet potato can also be broiled.)

3. Arrange the pepper strips and sweet potato slices on a platter or in a shallow bowl. Decorate with the herbs, sprinkle some salt and freshly ground black pepper over the vegetables, and drizzle with balsamic vinegar and any remaining oil.

4. Serve with crusty low G.I. rolls.

Serves 4 • Preparation time: 10 minutes • Cooking time: 25 minutes

Croutons

 low

CALORIES: 87
PROTEIN: 2G
FAT: 5G
CARBOHYDRATE: 8G
FIBER: 1G

4 slices stoneground, whole grain bread,
cut into 36 pieces per slice

2 tablespoons olive oil

2 tablespoons Parmesan cheese, grated

1 clove garlic, crushed

vegetable spray

1. Preheat oven to 400°F.
2. Toss cubes of bread in bowl with olive oil, grated cheese and garlic.
3. Spread out on baking sheet. Bake 10 minutes, turning once.
4. Cool before using.

Makes 2 cups

Serves 8 • Preparation time: 10 minutes • Cooking time: 10 minutes

dressings/sauces

Tomato and Olive Vinaigrette

 zero

CALORIES: 66
PROTEIN: 0G
FAT: 7G
CARBOHYDRATE: 0G
FIBER: 0G

4 tablespoons olive oil

1 small lemon, juice only

1 tablespoon white wine vinegar

1 clove garlic, crushed

1 teaspoon grainy mustard

1 tablespoon flat-leaf parsley, finely chopped

1 small, ripe plum tomato, finely diced

4 pitted kalamata olives, finely diced

1. Combine all ingredients in small screw-top jar. Shake well to combine.
2. Let stand 20 to 30 minutes before serving.

Makes 1 cup

Serves 8 • Preparation time: 10 minutes

Mediterranean Pasta Sauce

 low

CALORIES: 87
PROTEIN: 0G
FAT: 6G
CARBOHYDRATE: 7G
FIBER: 2G

¼ cup olive oil

1 large onion, chopped

1 medium green pepper, diced

2 tablespoons minced garlic

28-oz. can seeded tomatoes

12 large cured black olives, pitted and sliced

1 cup artichoke hearts, quartered

1. In a large saucepan, heat the oil gently, then add the onion, pepper and garlic. Sauté 2 minutes or until the onion becomes translucent.
2. Add the tomatoes and olives.
3. Bring to a boil, then simmer for 15 minutes.
4. Just before removing sauce from heat, add the artichoke hearts.
5. Serve over pasta.

Makes 5 cups

Serves 10 • Preparation time: 15 minutes • Cooking time: 20 minutes

CHAPTER 12

Pasta, Noodles and Grains

Vegetable and Sesame Noodle Stir-Fry

 low

CALORIES: 162
PROTEIN: 9G
FAT: 9G
CARBOHYDRATE: 42G
FIBER: 2G
OMEGA-3: ***

2 cups fresh linguine noodles

2 tablespoons sesame oil

1 cup snow peas

1 cup green pepper

1 cup baby corn, drained and thinly sliced

¼ cup shallots, thinly sliced

1 tablespoon fresh garlic, minced

1 teaspoon fresh ginger, minced

2 tablespoons teriyaki sauce

salt to taste

1. Place noodles in large bowl and cover with boiling water. Set aside.

2. Heat sesame oil in wok on low flame.

3. Wash snow peas and pepper, pat dry, and dice coarsely.

4. Increase heat. Add vegetables and spices (snow peas through ginger) and stir fry for 3 minutes.

5. Thoroughly drain noodles and add to wok. Drizzle teriyaki sauce and salt and toss well. Stir fry 1 minute. Serve immediately.

Serves 4 • Preparation time: 25 minutes • Cooking time: 4 minutes

Fresh Fettuccine with Scallops

 low

CALORIES: 157
PROTEIN: 10G
FAT: 4G
CARBOHYDRATE: 21G
FIBER: 2G
OMEGA-3: ***

2 9-oz. packages fresh fettuccine

24 sea scallops

4 cloves garlic, coarsely chopped

3 red chili peppers,
seeded and coarsely chopped

1 bunch flat leafed parsley, coarsely chopped

1 tablespoon extra virgin olive oil

salt and freshly ground black pepper

1. Cook the pasta in rapidly boiling salted water for 3 minutes.
2. Combine the chopped garlic, chilies and parsley in a small bowl.
3. Heat the olive oil in a heavy frying pan and add the scallops, cooking for 2 minutes, turning once only. Remove from the pan.
4. Add the garlic, chilies and parsley to the pan and heat through. Add the drained pasta, add a grind of salt and black pepper, toss and serve immediately, topped with the cooked scallops.

Serves 4–6 • Preparation time: 5 minutes • Cooking time: 10 minutes

Fettuccine with Vegetables and Sausage

Ⓖ low

CALORIES: 325
PROTEIN: 15G
FAT: 18G
CARBOHYDRATE: 41G
FIBER: 9G
OMEGA-3: *

12 ozs. spinach fettuccine

1 teaspoon olive oil

2 large onions, coarsely chopped

2 cloves garlic, coarsely chopped

4 stalks celery, thickly sliced (retain the young leaves for garnish)

1 large can (28 oz.) whole peeled tomatoes, undrained

3 tablespoons tomato paste

6 sprigs thyme or 1 teaspoon dried thyme

6 sprigs oregano or 1 teaspoon dried oregano

salt and freshly ground black pepper

½ cup capers

10 pitted black olives

4 sweet Italian sausages, sliced

1. Boil 3 quarts of salted water, add the fettuccine and stir until the water returns to a boil. Let boil, uncovered, until the pasta is cooked and "al dente."
2. Drain, toss a little oil through the pasta and keep warm.
3. Meanwhile, heat the olive oil over a moderate heat in a large heavy pan. Cook the onions and garlic for 3 minutes, stirring, then add the celery, undrained tomatoes, tomato paste, herbs, and seasonings, and simmer gently for 15 minutes.
4. Add the capers, olives and sliced sausages and simmer for a further 5 minutes.
5. Toss the sauce through the pasta and serve immediately, garnished with the small, young celery leaves.

Serves 4 • Preparation time: 5 minutes • Cooking time: 25 minutes

Grilled Vegetables and Beans with Pasta

 low

CALORIES: 362
PROTEIN: 14G
FAT: 7G
CARBOHYDRATE: 65G
FIBER: 11G
OMEGA-3: *

2 small Italian eggplants, cut in half lengthwise

2 large peppers, seeded and cut into thick strips

6 plum tomatoes, cut in half lengthwise

1 Spanish (red) onion, thickly sliced

4 cloves garlic, coarsely chopped

1 tablespoon olive oil

salt and freshly ground black pepper

1 15-oz. can light red kidney beans, drained

8 ozs. angel hair pasta

½ bunch basil leaves, torn

1. Prepare the vegetables.
2. Brush the BBQ grill with the olive oil, heat well and add all the prepared vegetables. Grind salt and pepper over the mixture and cook until the vegetables are golden brown, turning occasionally. Add the beans and toss through.
3. Meanwhile, boil 3 quarts of salted water and cook the pasta, uncovered, for about 4 to 5 minutes until "al dente." Drain.
4. On a large platter, arrange the pasta and vegetables, and scatter with torn basil leaves. Serve hot.

Serves 4 • Preparation time: 15 minutes • Cooking time: 15 minutes

Spaghetti with Steamed Greens

1 lb. spaghetti

4 large zucchini

12 snow peas, strings removed

1 cup (packed) baby spinach leaves

1 tablespoon lemon juice

2 tablespoons olive oil

1 clove garlic, crushed

salt and freshly ground black pepper

8 basil leaves, torn

1 tablespoon sesame oil

2 tablespoons toasted sesame seeds

1. Boil the spaghetti in plenty of lightly salted water for 13 minutes or until tender.

2. While spaghetti is cooking, wash the zucchini, and slice thinly lengthwise into long matchsticks. Wash and string the snow peas. Steam both until just softened and still bright green.

3. Mix together the lemon juice, olive oil, garlic and seasonings. Drain the spaghetti. Toss the vegetables, dressing, spinach and basil leaves through the spaghetti. Drizzle with sesame oil and sprinkle with toasted sesame seeds. Serve hot.

NOTE: To toast raw sesame seeds, simply add to a small heated frying pan and toss continually until they begin to turn a light golden brown. Remove immediately to prevent burning, and cool.

Serves 4–6 • Preparation time: 5 minutes • Cooking time: 13 minutes

Garlic Prawns, Pepper and Cilantro Pasta

 low

CALORIES: 382
PROTEIN: 25G
FAT: 11G
CARBOHYDRATE: 44G
FIBER: 1G
OMEGA-3: ***

12 ozs. spinach fettuccine

1 lb. giant tiger prawns

4 cloves garlic, finely sliced

¼ cup extra virgin olive oil

salt and freshly ground black pepper

2 large red or yellow peppers, seeded and thinly sliced

½ bunch fresh cilantro, coarsely chopped

1. Heat a large pot of salted water.
2. Preheat the grill to moderately high.
3. Meanwhile, shell and de-vein the prawns, leaving heads and tails on if desired. Toss with the sliced garlic and olive oil in a large bowl, and marinate for 10 minutes.
4. When water boils, add the pasta and cooked uncovered for about 11 minutes. Stir occasionally.
5. Grill the prawns for 2 minutes, coating them with the marinade, until cooked.
6. Grind salt and freshly ground black pepper over the prawns.
7. Drain the pasta and toss in 1 teaspoon of olive oil.
8. On a large serving platter combine the pasta, prawns, pepper strips and chopped cilantro.
9. Serve hot with crusty low G.I. bread.

Serves 4–6 • Preparation time: 8 minutes • Cooking time: 11 minutes

Spiral Noodles with Smoked Turkey and Pine Nuts

low

CALORIES: 359
PROTEIN: 17G
FAT: 20G
CARBOHYDRATE: 29G
FIBER: 4G
OMEGA-3: *

8 ozs. spinach fettuccine

1 teaspoon salt

2 tablespoons pine nuts

2 small chili peppers, seeded and finely sliced

8 ozs. smoked turkey breast

½ bunch flat leafed parsley, finely chopped

Dressing

4 tablespoons olive oil

4 tablespoons balsamic vinegar

1 clove garlic, crushed

salt and freshly ground black pepper

1. Boil 4 quarts of salted water and cook the noodles until tender. Refresh under cold running water.
2. Meanwhile, dry roast the pine nuts in a heavy frying pan, stirring constantly, until golden brown.
3. Finely slice the chilies and turkey breast.
4. Place all the dressing ingredients in a lidded jar and shake to combine.
5. Combine the noodles, pine nuts, chilies and turkey breast on a large platter, sprinkle with chopped parsley and pour the dressing over.

Serves 6 • Preparation time: 5 minutes • Cooking time: 10 minutes

Marinated BBQ Chicken Noodle Salad

 low

CALORIES: 336
PROTEIN: 36G
FAT: 2G
CARBOHYDRATE: 42G
FIBER: 3G
OMEGA-3: ***

¼ teaspoon chili flakes or
1 whole dried chili, finely chopped
1 tablespoon canola oil
2 cloves garlic, finely chopped
2 strips lemon zest, finely chopped
1 lb. chicken tenders
8 ozs. angel hair pasta
½ bunch fresh cilantro, coarsely chopped

1. Combine the chili, oil, garlic, lemon zest and chicken pieces in a bowl and marinate for 15 minutes.
2. Preheat the grill. Cook the chicken until golden brown, about 6 minutes. Cut into bite-size cubes (about 1").
3. Meanwhile, cook the pasta in plenty of boiling, salted water for 10 minutes.
4. Drain and toss the chicken pieces and chopped cilantro through the noodles, and serve immediately.

Serves 4 • Preparation time: 20 minutes • Cooking time: 10 minutes

Tofu Chicken with Snow Peas and Rice Noodles

 low

CALORIES: 530
PROTEIN: 24G
FAT: 8G
CARBOHYDRATE: 40G
FIBER: 6G
OMEGA-3: **

1 lb. chicken tenderloins, sliced into narrow strips
2 cloves garlic, finely chopped
1 tablespoon sesame oil
¼ cup vegetable or chicken stock
10 ozs. broccoli florets
3 ozs. snow peas, strings removed
5 4½-oz. packages rice noodles, soaked in boiling water
1 tablespoon toasted sesame seeds

Marinade

3 tablespoons light soy sauce
1 tablespoon hoisin sauce
1 tablespoon oyster sauce
1 tablespoon rice wine (mirin)
5 ozs. firm tofu, diced

1. Combine the marinade ingredients in a large mixing bowl and toss the tofu cubes through the mixture.
2. Heat the sesame oil in a large wok and stir-fry the chicken and garlic for 3 minutes. Remove and set aside.
3. Add the stock and broccoli florets, cover and simmer for 3 minutes. Add the snow peas and cook a further minute.
4. Add the marinade and tofu, chicken and drained noodles. Toss to warm noodles. Serve hot, sprinkled with toasted sesame seeds.

Serves 6–8 • Preparation time: 15 minutes • Cooking time: 10 minutes

Butter Bean, Pepper and Shrimp Pilaf

(G) low

CALORIES: 275
PROTEIN: 24G
FAT: 4G
CARBOHYDRATE: 39G
FIBER: 6G
OMEGA-3: ***

1 tablespoon canola oil

1 cup Basmati rice

1 large onion, chopped

1 teaspoon turmeric or ginger

2 cloves garlic, chopped

1 large green pepper, seeded and diced

½ can (about 13 ozs.) whole
peeled tomatoes, undrained

2 cups chicken or vegetable stock

salt and freshly ground black pepper

1 15.5-oz. can butter beans, drained

1 red chili, seeded and finely sliced

2 lbs. medium green shrimp, shelled and de-veined*

½ bunch fresh cilantro, coarsely chopped

1. Heat the oil in a large, heavy frying pan and add the rice, onion and turmeric or ginger. Stir the rice for 3 minutes before adding the garlic, pepper, tomatoes and juice, stock and salt and pepper.
2. Cover the pan with a tight-fitting lid and simmer for 20 minutes, until the rice absorbs most of the stock.
3. Gently stir the butter beans, chili and shrimp through the mixture and cook, covered, for another 3 minutes.
4. Taste for seasoning, stir through the cilantro and serve immediately.

*NOTE: This recipe can also be made with scallops.

Serves 4–6 • Preparation time: 10 minutes • Cooking time: 30 minutes

Chicken, Fennel and Lemon Paella

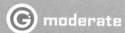 **moderate**

CALORIES: 312
PROTEIN: 18G
FAT: 8G
CARBOHYDRATE: 43G
FIBER: 3 G
OMEGA-3: *

1 tablespoon olive oil

1 medium bulb fennel (anise), finely sliced

1 small onion, finely sliced

2 cloves garlic, coarsely chopped

1 lb. chicken tenders

2 cups Basmati rice, uncooked

salt and freshly ground black pepper

4 cups chicken stock, boiling

½ bunch fresh dill, finely chopped (⅓ cup)

juice and zest of ½ lemon

1 cup fresh Parmesan cheese, shaved

a few sprigs of dill for decoration

1. Preheat the oven to 400°F.
2. Heat the oil in a large, ovenproof, heavy frying pan. Add the fennel, onion and garlic, and cook until they become opaque, approx. 2 minutes. Remove and set aside.
3. Add the tenders and cook for 3 to 4 minutes, until just cooked through. Remove and set aside.
4. Stir in the rice and cook for 2 minutes. Season.
5. Heat the chicken stock in a saucepan to boiling, then pour it into the frying pan. Stir the stock through the rice, and add the fennel, onion, garlic, chopped dill, and lemon juice and zest.
6. Place the pan in the oven and cook, uncovered, for 20 minutes.
7. Add the chicken tenderloins and Parmesan and gently fork them through the rice.
8. Serve immediately, decorated with sprigs of dill.

Serves 6–8 • Preparation time: 10 minutes • Cooking time: 35 minutes

Stuffed Eggplant

low

CALORIES: 284
PROTEIN: 12G
FAT: 16G
CARBOHYDRATE: 22G
FIBER: 8G
OMEGA-3: *

½ cup pearl barley, uncooked

3 cups water

2 medium-size eggplants, halved lengthwise

2 medium ripe tomatoes, finely diced

6 shallots, finely sliced

2 sprigs fresh oregano,
or 1 teaspoon dried oregano

2 sprigs fresh marjoram, or 1 teaspoon dried marjoram

2 sprigs fresh thyme, or 1 teaspoon dried thyme

2 tablespoons olive oil

2 large cloves garlic, finely chopped

1 heaping cup Parmesan cheese, grated

salt and freshly ground black pepper

few extra sprigs fresh oregano, marjoram or thyme for garnish

1. Preheat the oven to 350°F.
2. Simmer the pearl barley, covered, in the water for 30 minutes.
3. Meanwhile, scoop out the flesh of the eggplants, leaving a ½" shell. Sprinkle the shell with salt and turn upside down on paper towels to drain off the bitter juices. Dice the eggplant flesh.
4. Combine the diced tomatoes, sliced shallots and chopped herbs.
5. Heat the olive oil in a large, heavy frying pan and add the chopped garlic and diced eggplant. Sauté until the eggplant browns. Fold through the tomato mixture and drained barley, and stir in the Parmesan cheese. Season with salt and freshly ground black pepper.
6. Rinse the eggplant shells out with cold water and pat dry. Fill with the stuffing and bake for 30 minutes.
7. Garnish with sprigs of fresh herbs and serve hot.

Serves 4 • Preparation time: 10 minutes • Cooking time: 40 minutes

Roasted Sweet Potato, Garlic and Rosemary Pilaf

G moderate

CALORIES: 444
PROTEIN: 12G
FAT: 10G
CARBOHYDRATE: 76G
FIBER: 5G
OMEGA-3: *

2 lbs. sweet potato, peeled and cubed
8 cloves garlic, peeled and halved
3 sprigs fresh rosemary
1 tablespoon olive oil
4 cups chicken or vegetable stock, hot
1 tablespoon olive oil
2 cups Basmati rice, uncooked
salt and freshly ground black pepper
6 extra sprigs fresh rosemary
1 cup freshly grated Parmesan cheese

1. Preheat the oven to 400°F.
2. Place the cubed sweet potato, garlic cloves and sprigs of rosemary in a baking tray, and sprinkle with the olive oil.
3. Roast the sweet potato until just golden, approx. 20 minutes. Remove from the oven.
4. Heat the chicken stock to boiling point.
5. Heat the olive oil in a large, heavy saucepan and stir in the rice. Coat the rice with oil and cook for 2 minutes, stirring.
6. Add the sweet potato and garlic, and season with salt and pepper. Discard the rosemary sprigs. Add the hot chicken stock and turn the heat down to simmering.
7. Cover and cook gently for 15 minutes, until all the stock is absorbed and the rice is cooked through. Stir the Parmesan through.
8. Turn the pilaf into 6 large pasta bowls, and decorate each with a fresh rosemary sprig.

Serves 6 • Preparation time: 10 minutes • Cooking time: 40 minutes

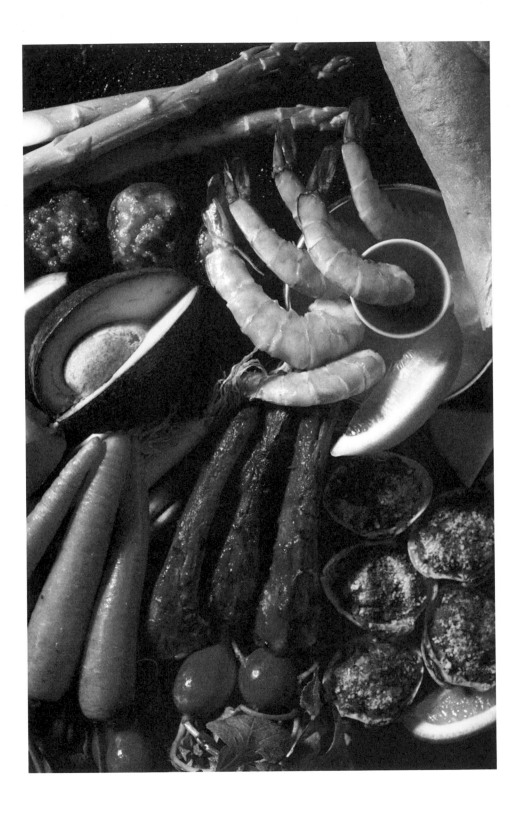

CHAPTER 13

Entrées and Accompaniments

Chickpea Burgers

 low

CALORIES: 191
PROTEIN: 8G
FAT: 2G
CARBOHYDRATE: 36G
FIBER: 5 G

19-oz. can chickpeas, drained

2 cups boiling potatoes, cooked and mashed

¹/₄ cup egg substitute

¹/₃ cup shallots

1 clove fresh garlic

1 small lemon, juice only

2 tablespoons fresh mint, coarsely chopped

vegetable spray

1. Place all ingredients in blender, process 1 minute.
2. Coat skillet with vegetable spray. Scoop ¹/₂ cup of mixture onto skillet to form patty, pressing down slightly with back of fork.
3. Repeat with another 3 or 4 scoops, depending on skillet size.
4. Cook 5 minutes per side. Serve hot or cold.

Makes 10

Serves 5 • Preparation time: 10 minutes • Cooking time: 10 minutes

Salmon and Butter Bean Salad

G low

CALORIES: 233
PROTEIN: 18G
FAT: 7G
CARBOHYDRATE: 29G
FIBER: 7G
OMEGA-3: ****

6 ozs. canned salmon, drained

1 15.5-oz. can butter beans, drained

½ small cucumber, sliced

½ red onion, diced

1 tablespoon olive oil

1 tablespoon lemon juice

1 clove garlic, minced

black pepper to taste

1. Place salmon in medium mixing bowl. Break into small chunks.
2. Add remaining ingredients (butter beans through pepper) and mix well. Serve cold.

Serves 3 • Preparation time: 10 minutes

The Glucose Revolution Life Plan

Sardine Toast Topper

CALORIES: 123
PROTEIN: 6G
FAT: 10G
CARBOHYDRATE: 3G
FIBER: 0G
OMEGA-3: *****

$4\frac{1}{4}$-oz.-can sardines, packed in water, drained

1 clove garlic, crushed

$1\frac{1}{2}$ tablespoon capers, drained

10 pitted black olives

½ bunch flat-leafed parsley, chopped

1 tablespoon red wine vinegar

1 tablespoon olive oil

1. Place all ingredients in food processor.
2. Process until just combined.
3. Serve as a spread on toasted low G.I. bread

Makes ¾ cup

Serves 3 • Preparation time: 5 minutes

Tuna-Veggie Toss

 low

CALORIES: 99
PROTEIN: 9G
FAT: 3G
CARBOHYDRATE: 10G
FIBER: 2G
OMEGA-3: ***

2 cups medium pasta shells, uncooked
6-oz. can tuna, packed in water, drained
1 clove garlic, minced
black pepper to taste
1 1/2 tablespoons fresh parsley, finely chopped
1 1/2 tablespoons fresh basil, finely chopped,
or 1 1/2 teaspoons dried
1 tablespoon olive oil
2 cups cooked, reheated vegetables, such as
zucchini, mushrooms, broccoli, peppers

1. Cook pasta according to package directions. Remember not to overcook.
2. Meanwhile, mix all remaining ingredients in large serving dish.
3. Drain pasta and add to tuna-vegetable mixture. Toss well, and serve immediately.

Makes 6 cups

*NOTE: You can replace leftover vegetables with freshly cooked.

NOTE: To leftover or fresh boiled small pasta (for example, bows or spirals) add a can of drained tuna (or salmon), crushed garlic, black pepper, chopped fresh herbs such as parsley and basil, and a drizzle of olive oil. Mix in some reheated leftover vegetables such as zucchini, mushroom, broccoli or pepper.

Serves 6 • Preparation time: 10 minutes • Cooking time: Depends on pasta package directions.

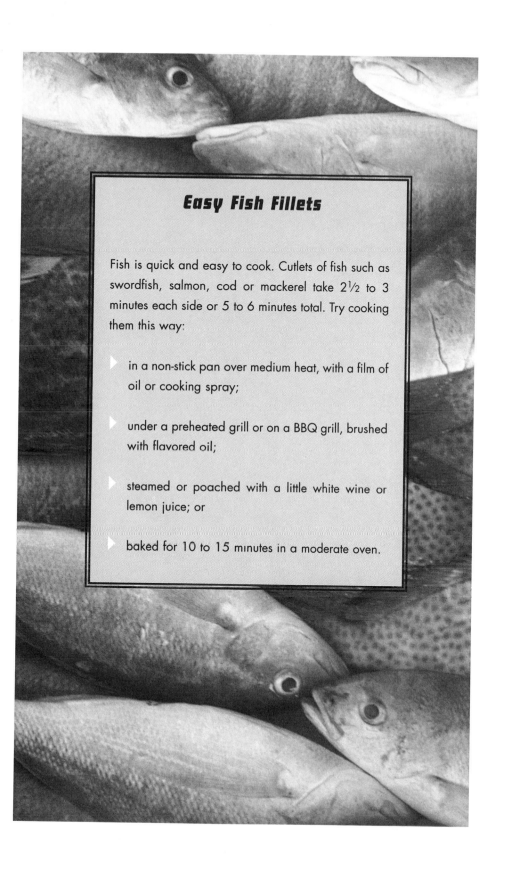

Easy Fish Fillets

Fish is quick and easy to cook. Cutlets of fish such as swordfish, salmon, cod or mackerel take 2½ to 3 minutes each side or 5 to 6 minutes total. Try cooking them this way:

- in a non-stick pan over medium heat, with a film of oil or cooking spray;

- under a preheated grill or on a BBQ grill, brushed with flavored oil;

- steamed or poached with a little white wine or lemon juice; or

- baked for 10 to 15 minutes in a moderate oven.

Mediterranean Beef Stew

1 tablespoon olive oil

1 large onion, thinly sliced

2 lbs. eye round beef, cut into 1-inch cubes

$\frac{1}{2}$ cup red wine

salt and pepper to taste

1 cup crushed tomatoes

1 large bay leaf

1 cup dried porcini mushrooms, rehydrated in 1 cup warm water

1 lb. baby carrots, halved

1 teaspoon fresh thyme, finely chopped

1$\frac{1}{2}$ tablespoon fresh parsley, finely chopped

1. Heat oil in large skillet. Add onion and sauté for 2 minutes.
2. Add beef cubes to skillet. Sauté 3 minutes or until all sides are browned.
3. Add wine, salt and pepper.
4. Add tomatoes and bay leaf. Bring to a boil, then simmer for 1 hour.
5. Remove mushrooms from water. DO NOT THROW WATER AWAY. Strain it, and add to stew mixture.
6. Add carrots and herbs and mix well. Simmer for 30 minutes.
7. Serve over noodles or rice.

Makes 6 cups

Serves 6 • Preparation time: 20 minutes • Cooking time: About 1 $\frac{1}{2}$ hours

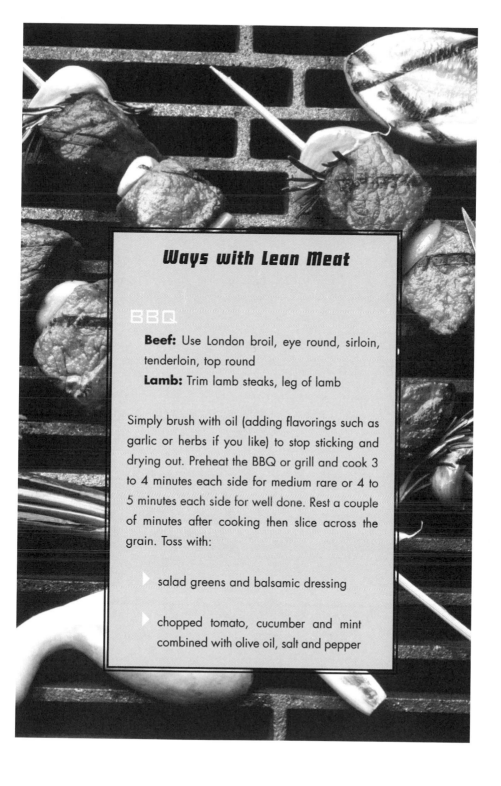

Ways with Lean Meat

BBQ

Beef: Use London broil, eye round, sirloin, tenderloin, top round

Lamb: Trim lamb steaks, leg of lamb

Simply brush with oil (adding flavorings such as garlic or herbs if you like) to stop sticking and drying out. Preheat the BBQ or grill and cook 3 to 4 minutes each side for medium rare or 4 to 5 minutes each side for well done. Rest a couple of minutes after cooking then slice across the grain. Toss with:

▸ salad greens and balsamic dressing

▸ chopped tomato, cucumber and mint combined with olive oil, salt and pepper

Pork Fillet with Spiced Pears and Basmati Rice

low

CALORIES: 353
PROTEIN: 22G
FAT: 2G
CARBOHYDRATE: 59G
FIBER: 6G
OMEGA-3: *

2 teaspoons olive oil

1 large onion, diced

2 cloves garlic, finely chopped

2 medium sweet potatoes, diced

1 cup Basmati rice, uncooked

1½ cups chicken stock

salt and freshly ground black pepper

4 Bosc pears, peeled, cored and quartered

1 cinnamon stick

4 whole cloves

2 strips of lemon zest

¼ cup sugar

1 teaspoon olive oil

1 clove garlic, finely chopped

1 lb. pork fillets, center loin

⅓ cup dry white wine

salt and freshly ground black pepper

½ bunch chives for garnish

Serves 4–6 • Preparation time: 10 minutes • Cooking time: 45 minutes

1. Heat the oil in a large saucepan with a tight-fitting lid over a moderate heat. Add the onion, garlic and diced sweet potato and cook for 3 minutes, stirring.
2. Add the rice and cook for a further 3 minutes, stirring to coat the ingredients in oil and partially cook.
3. Pour in the chicken stock, season with salt and pepper, cover with a tight-fitting lid and turn the heat down to low. Simmer very gently for 15 minutes, until all the stock is absorbed and the rice is cooked.
4. Meanwhile, place the pears, cinnamon stick, cloves, lemon zest and sugar in a large saucepan and cover with 1 quart of water. Bring to a boil, then turn the heat down to gently simmer the pears, uncovered, for 20 minutes.
5. Heat the 1 teaspoon of oil in a heavy frying pan and brown the pork fillets on all sides. Continue to cook the fillets over a moderate heat for approx. 15 minutes, until just cooked through. Remove the fillets from the pan and keep warm.
6. Add the garlic and white wine to the pan juices and simmer, stirring the sauce, for about 3 minutes. Season with salt and pepper.
7. Slice the pork fillets diagonally.
8. To assemble, place mounds of Basmati rice on warmed plates, top with slices of pork and pour the reduction sauce over the top. Garnish with whole chives. Fan the pear slices on the plate and pour a little juice over the top.
9. Serve hot, accompanied by steamed baby carrots.

Carrot and Thyme Quiche

 low

CALORIES: 209
PROTEIN: 8G
FAT: 15G
CARBOHYDRATE: 11G
FIBER: 6G
OMEGA-3: ***

2 lbs. carrots, peeled and grated

1 large onion, peeled and grated

2 cloves garlic, grated or finely chopped

2½ ozs. low fat cheddar cheese, grated

⅓ cup canola oil

3 eggs, lightly beaten

1 teaspoon ground nutmeg

salt and freshly ground pepper

1 tablespoon fresh thyme leaves, or 1 teaspoon dried

½ cup self-raising flour

1. Preheat the oven to 350°F.

2. Lightly oil a 12-inch round shallow quiche or pie dish.

3. Grate the carrots, onion, garlic and cheese (using the grating disc of your food processor makes this step quick and easy).

4. In a large mixing bowl beat together the oil, eggs, nutmeg, salt and pepper, and thyme leaves. Stir in the flour until combined, then add the carrots, onion, garlic and cheese.

5. Spoon into the prepared dish and bake for 45 minutes, until golden brown and cooked through.

Serves 6–8 • Preparation time: 15 minutes • Cooking time: 45 minutes

Roast Chicken with Apricot and Almond Stuffing

 low

CALORIES: 365
PROTEIN: 40G
FAT: 16G
CARBOHYDRATE: 16G
FIBER: 4G
OMEGA-3: ***

1 chicken (about 3-3½ lbs.), skin and visible fat removed, washed

½ cup quick-cook barley

12 dried apricots, coarsely chopped

⅓ cup unblanched almonds, coarsely chopped

½ bunch flat leafed parsley, coarsely chopped

juice and zest of ½ lemon

1 egg, lightly beaten

salt and freshly ground black pepper

1 tablespoon olive oil

2 cups chicken (or vegetable) stock

1. Preheat the oven to 350°F.
2. In a bowl, combine the uncooked barley, chopped apricots, almonds and parsley, juice and zest of lemon, lightly beaten egg, and season with salt and pepper.
3. Stuff the chicken and place, breast side up, in a lightly oiled baking dish. Tie the legs together with string and rub the chicken with the remaining olive oil. Pour the stock into the dish.
4. Cover the dish with foil and place in the oven. Bake for one hour, then remove the foil and bake a further 30 minutes, basting the chicken with the stock to brown it up and keep it moist.
5. Remove the chicken from the dish and discard the string. Keep the chicken warm while making the sauce.
6. Make a reduction sauce by simmering the stock in the baking dish over a moderate heat to reduce by half. Season with salt and pepper and strain. Serve hot.

Serves 6 • Preparation time: 10 minutes • Cooking time: 1½ hours

Thai Chicken Curry

G moderate

CALORIES: 401
PROTEIN: 33G
FAT: 11G
CARBOHYDRATE: 43G
FIBER: 4G
OMEGA-3: **

2 lbs. chicken breasts or thigh fillets,
sliced thinly, fat removed
2 large onions, finely chopped
1 tablespoon canola oil
2 tablespoons green curry paste
1 stalk lemongrass
1½ cups chicken stock
7 ozs. low fat (light) coconut milk
7 ozs. water
2 green chilies, finely sliced
8 ozs. green beans, diagonally sliced
1 bunch fresh cilantro, coarsely chopped
2 cups Basmati rice, uncooked
6 quarts water

1. Heat the oil in a large heavy frying pan and add the onions. Cook gently for 5 minutes, then add the curry paste and cook for 2 minutes, stirring.
2. Crush the lemongrass stalk and add to the pan. Add the chicken stock, coconut milk and water and simmer for 10 minutes to reduce the liquid.
3. Add chilies and chicken. Simmer gently until the chicken is tender.
4. Bring the water to a boil and slowly pour in the rice, stirring until the water returns to a boil. Boil for 11 minutes, then drain immediately. While the rice is cooking, steam the green beans separately until just tender.
5. Remove the lemongrass from the curry, add the beans and chopped cilantro.
6. Serve on a bed of hot Basmati rice with a garnish of cilantro.

Serves 6–8 • Preparation time: 5 minutes • Cooking time: 17 minutes

Rack of Lamb with Lemon and Rosemary on Potato-Garlic Mash

 zero

CALORIES: 178
PROTEIN: 17G
FAT: 12G
CARBOHYDRATE: NEG
FIBER: NEG
OMEGA-3: *

2 racks of lamb, 6 chops each

3 cloves garlic

6 sprigs fresh rosemary

zest of 1 lemon

freshly ground black pepper

2 tablespoons olive oil

6 sprigs fresh rosemary for garnish

Sweet Potato, Potato and Garlic Mash (page 205)

1. Preheat the oven to 400°C.
2. Trim the racks of lamb with a small knife, removing all visible fat. Peel and halve the cloves of garlic, and break the rosemary sprigs into smaller sprigs. Remove the zest from the lemon with a zester or vegetable peeler.
3. Cut a tunnel between the bone and the meat, and fill with garlic halves, lemon zest and a couple of rosemary sprigs.
4. Pierce the lamb and insert sprigs of rosemary over the surface of the rack.
5. Place the racks in a baking dish, grind a little black pepper over them and sprinkle with olive oil.
6. Bake for 35 to 40 minutes in the preheated oven until cooked through but slightly pink. (If using a meat thermometer, internal temperature should be between 175° and 182°F.)
7. Let the lamb rest for 5 minutes in a warm place before cutting into cutlets.
8. Serve on a bed of hot Sweet Potato, Potato and Garlic Mash. Decorate with a sprig of fresh rosemary.

Serves 6 • Preparation time: 10 minutes • Cooking time: 40 minutes

Red Pepper with Grilled Vegetables and Giant Tiger Prawns

 low

CALORIES: 243
PROTEIN: 13G
FAT: 14G
CARBOHYDRATE: 18G
FIBER: 6G
OMEGA-3: **

2 bunches fresh basil

²/₃ cup unblanched whole almonds, coarsely chopped

4 cloves garlic, peeled

¼ cup extra virgin olive oil

salt and freshly ground black pepper

4 medium-sized red peppers

8 Italian eggplants

12 small plum tomatoes

2 tablespoons olive oil

4 cloves garlic, finely chopped

salt and freshly ground black pepper

1 cup penne pasta, uncooked

16 giant tiger prawns, shelled and de-veined (tails optional)

Serves 8 • Preparation time: 20 minutes • Cooking time: 30 minutes

1. Preheat the oven to 350°F. Also preheat the grill.
2. Make a pesto with 1 1/2 bunches of basil leaves. First use a food processor to process the almonds coarsely. Add the garlic, olive oil, salt and freshly ground black pepper and remaining basil leaves, and process to a coarse puree.
3. Cut the peppers in half lengthwise. Remove the seeds and white membrane from the inside cavities. Halve the eggplant lengthwise. Halve the plum tomatoes lengthwise and remove seeds.
4. Combine the olive oil, chopped garlic, salt and freshly ground black pepper. Use half the mixture to brush the tomatoes. Top them with the remaining 1/2 bunch of basil leaves, shredded. Place on an oven tray and bake for 30 minutes in the preheated oven.
5. Place the pepper halves, cut side down, on a baking tray and bake in the oven until they soften but do not lose shape. Remove and pat dry with paper kitchen towel. Take care to keep them from breaking.
6. Boil 4 quarts of salted water and cook the penne for 9–11 minutes.
7 While the pasta is cooking, brush the halved eggplant and the prawns with the remaining garlic and olive oil mixture, and grill them until tender (about 3 minutes).
8. Drain the pasta and toss with 1-2 tablespoons olive oil.
9. To assemble, fill the pepper shells with the roasted tomatoes and baked basil leaves, pasta, eggplant halves and grilled prawns. Top with a large dollop of pesto.

Grilled Blue-Eye Cod
with Warm Bean Salad

(G) low

CALORIES: 309
PROTEIN: 33G
FAT: 10G
CARBOHYDRATE: 21G
FIBER: 11G
OMEGA-3: ****

2 15.5-oz. cans light red kidney beans,
½ cup liquid reserved

1 cup chicken or vegetable stock

3 cloves garlic, crushed

2 large ripe tomatoes, coarsely chopped

2 bunches arugula, washed and coarsely chopped

1 bunch shallots, finely sliced

¼ bunch flat leafed parsley, finely chopped

3 tablespoons lemon juice

1 tablespoon olive oil

4 4-oz. blue-eye cod fillets

freshly ground black pepper

extra arugula leaves for garnish

1. In a bowl, mash ½ cup of beans with a little reserved liquid from the can.
2. Place the mashed beans, remaining whole beans, chicken stock, garlic, tomatoes, chopped arugula, sliced shallots, chopped parsley, lemon juice, salt and pepper in a large saucepan.
3. Warm the bean mixture, covered, over a low heat for approx. 10 minutes, while cooking the cod.
4. Preheat the BBQ grill or grill plate on the stove and brush with olive oil. Grind black pepper over the cod cutlets and cook for approximately 8 minutes, turning once only.
5. Serve the warm bean salad as a bed for the blue eye cod fillets, and garnish with extra arugula leaves.

Serves 4 • Preparation time: 10 minutes • Cooking time: 8 minutes

Deep Sea Perch* on Roasted Vegetables

CALORIES: 239
PROTEIN: 29G
FAT: 10G
CARBOHYDRATE: 7G
FIBER: 5G
OMEGA-3: ****

6 5-oz. deep sea perch fillets

1 tablespoon olive oil

3 medium zucchini, thickly sliced

6 ripe medium tomatoes, quartered and seeded

2 medium red onions, cut into wedges

1 large red pepper, thickly sliced

1 large green pepper, thickly sliced

4 large cloves garlic, coarsely chopped

8 sprigs fresh thyme or 2 tablespoons dried thyme leaves

2 tablespoons olive oil

salt and freshly ground black pepper

½ bunch fresh basil, leaves finely sliced

3 tablespoons balsamic vinegar

1. Preheat the oven to 500°F
2. Season the deep sea perch fillets with freshly ground black pepper, and brush with a little olive oil.
3. In a large baking dish, combine the prepared vegetables, garlic, thyme and olive oil, and spread in one layer. Grind salt and pepper over the vegetables.
4. Bake the vegetables in the preheated oven for 18–20 minutes, stirring occasionally. Arrange the fillets over the vegetables and roast for 6–9 minutes.
5. Transfer the fillets carefully to a warm plate and cover.
6. Arrange the vegetables on 6 warm plates and sprinkle with the basil leaves and a drizzle of balsamic vinegar. Top with the fillets and serve immediately with Basmati rice.

* **Note:** You can also use trout or carp for this recipe.

Serves 6 • Preparation time: 15 minutes • Cooking time: 30 minutes

Seared Tuna with Red Pepper Coulis

ⓖ moderate

CALORIES: 439
PROTEIN: 42G
FAT: 9G
CARBOHYDRATE: 48G
FIBER: 5G
OMEGA-3: *****

Coulis

4 large bright red peppers

1 large can (28 oz.) whole peeled tomatoes, drained and seeded

salt and freshly ground black pepper

6 tuna steaks (about 6 ozs. each)

2 tablespoons olive oil, divided

1½ cups Basmati rice, uncooked

4 cloves garlic, peeled and halved

1 lemon, juice and zest only

1. Rinse the tuna steaks and pat the tuna steaks with paper towels until dry. Brush them with 1 tablespoon olive oil. Set aside.

2. To make the coulis, halve and seed the peppers. Bake, broil or grill them, skin side up, until black and blistered. Place in a paper bag and let cool before removing skin. Puree with tomatoes in a food processor. Season with salt and pepper. Transfer coulis to a small sauce pan and keep warm.

3. Bring a large pot of salted water to a boil and cook the rice for 11 minutes.

4. In the meantime, preheat a large, heavy frying pan, then add the remaining olive oil. Toss in the garlic and heat through.

Serves 6 • Preparation time: 10 minutes • Cooking time: 35 minutes

5. Add the prepared tuna steaks, sear each side quickly, reduce to medium flame, and leave them, unturned, for 6 to 8 minutes, until cooked through.

6. Drain the rice when cooked and transfer to a serving platter. Keep warm.

7. Arrange the tuna on the bed of rice. Keep warm.

8. Remove garlic from pan. Add lemon juice to pan juice and heat through. Season with salt and pepper.

9. Pour juices over the tuna and add lemon zest for garnish.

10. Spoon the red pepper coulis around the serving platter and serve immediately.

*NOTE: You may grill the tuna steaks if you prefer.

Cod Fillets with Sun-dried Tomato Marinade

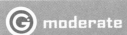 **moderate**

CALORIES: 281
PROTEIN: 34G
FAT: 12G
CARBOHYDRATE: 11G
FIBER: 3G
OMEGA-3: ****

1 cup sun-dried tomatoes in oil (reserve the oil)

2 cloves garlic, peeled and coarsely chopped

1 lemon, juice and zest only

freshly ground black pepper

2 lbs. cod fillets

flat-leafed parsley for garnish

1. Place the drained sun-dried tomatoes, $^1/_4$ cup of the reserved oil, garlic cloves, lemon juice, zest and pepper in the food processor, and blend to a smooth consistency.
2. Place the cod fillets in a shallow casserole dish, spread the marinade over, cover with foil and marinate for 30 minutes.
3. Preheat the oven to 350°F.
4. Bake the fillets, covered, until just cooked through (approx. 15 minutes). Remove from the oven and serve on a bed of steamed Basmati rice, with the marinade spooned over the top. Decorate with a few sprigs of flat leafed parsley.

Serves 6 • Preparation time: 35 minutes • Cooking time: 15 minutes

The Glucose Revolution Life Plan

Mediterranean Lasagna

CALORIES: 268
PROTEIN: 21G
FAT: 10G
CARBOHYDRATE: 24G
FIBER: 6G
OMEGA-3: *

1 tablespoon olive oil

1 lb. ground beef, lean

2 onions, chopped

4 cloves garlic, chopped

1 large can (28 oz.) whole peeled tomatoes

1/2 cup tomato paste

1 cup water

1/2 bunch fresh oregano, chopped

2 eggplants, cut into 1-inch slices

1 tablespoon olive oil

8 ozs. frozen chopped leaf spinach, thawed

1 teaspoon nutmeg

5 sheets large instant lasagna pasta

3 ozs. low fat cheddar cheese, grated

salt and freshly ground black pepper

1. Preheat the oven to 350°C.
2. Heat the oil in a large heavy saucepan over moderate heat. Add the onions and garlic and cook, stirring occasionally, for 3 minutes.
3. Add the chopped meat and cook until the meat turns brown, then add the tomatoes, tomato paste and water. Season with salt and pepper and add the chopped oregano. Cook for 30 minutes, stirring occasionally.
4. Brush the eggplant slices with oil and grill or broil until browned on each side.
5. Using a rectangular casserole dish (approx. 9" x 13"), layer the ingredients. Start with half the meat sauce, then 2½ sheets of lasagna, half the eggplant slices, all the spinach sprinkled with nutmeg, salt and pepper, 2½ sheets lasagna pasta, eggplant slices, meat sauce and grated cheese.
6. Bake for 40–45 minutes. Serve with a crisp green salad.

Serves 6–8 • Preparation time: 15 minutes • Cooking time: 75 minutes

Seared Atlantic Salmon Fillets with White Bean Puree

 low

CALORIES: 307
PROTEIN: 43G
FAT: 11G
CARBOHYDRATE: 9G
FIBER: 6G
OMEGA-3: *****

4 Atlantic salmon fillets, trimmed and boned

1 tablespoon olive oil

2 cloves garlic, halved

White bean puree

1 15.5-oz. can cannellini beans, drained

2 cloves garlic, crushed

1½ tablespoons lemon juice

4 sprigs fresh thyme leaves
or 1 tablespoon dried thyme

2 teaspoons olive oil

salt and freshly ground black pepper

1 bunch arugula

1. Preheat the hotplate of the BBQ or a heavy frying pan.
2. Using a food processor (or mash by hand), process the drained beans, garlic, lemon juice, thyme, olive oil, salt and pepper to a smooth, soft puree. Place in an ovenproof or microwave bowl, cover and warm through in a low oven or microwave.
3. To cook the Atlantic salmon fillets, heat the oil with the garlic cloves for 1 minute on the hotplate. Add the salmon fillets and cook for approximately 5 to 8 minutes, turning once only.
4. Place a large spoonful of cannellini bean puree in the center of heated plates, arrange arugula on top, and finish with the cooked fillets.
5. Drizzle a little extra oil around the plate and serve immediately.

Serves 4 • Preparation time: 10 minutes • Cooking time: 5–8 minutes

Grilled Garlic Potatoes and Sweet Potatoes

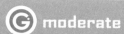 moderate

CALORIES: 226
PROTEIN: 4G
FAT: 10G
CARBOHYDRATE: 29G
FIBER: 3G

2 lbs. red potatoes

2 lbs. sweet potatoes

6 cloves garlic, coarsely chopped

1 sprig fresh rosemary

or 1 tablespoon dried rosemary

⅓ cup extra virgin olive oil

salt and freshly ground black pepper

a few extra sprigs rosemary for garnish

1. Peel the potatoes and sweet potatoes, and parboil in plenty of boiling salted water. Drain and set aside.
2. Preheat a lightly oiled grill or large heavy frying pan.
3. Mix the chopped garlic, rosemary, oil and seasonings together in a large mixing bowl. Cut the vegetables into large chunks and toss in the garlic oil.
4. Cook on the grill or in the frying pan until golden brown and crisp.
5. Serve hot in a large bowl with sprigs of fresh rosemary for garnish.

Serves 6–8 • Preparation time: 10 minutes • Cooking time: 20 minutes

Chickpea, Tomato and Eggplant

G low

CALORIES: 137
PROTEIN: 5G
FAT: 6G
CARBOHYDRATE: 15G
FIBER: 6G

1 15-oz. can chickpeas, drained

6 Italian eggplants

2 large onions

4 cloves garlic, peeled

2 tablespoons olive oil

½ teaspoon ground cumin

½ teaspoon ground cinnamon

½ teaspoon ground coriander

salt and freshly ground black pepper

2 large cans (28 oz.) whole peeled tomatoes, undrained

1. Drain the chickpeas, rinse well and set aside.
2. Dice the eggplants and onions, and finely chop the garlic.
3. Heat the olive oil in a large heavy frying pan, and gently cook the eggplants, onions, garlic and spices over a moderate heat for 10 minutes, stirring occasionally.
4. Season with salt and pepper, and add the undrained tomatoes, breaking them up with a wooden spoon. Add the drained chickpeas, cover and simmer for 20 minutes.
5. Serve warm with low G.I. crusty bread as an entrée, or as a side dish to the main course.

Serves 8 • Preparation time: 5 minutes • Cooking time: 30 minutes

Sweet Potato, Potato and Garlic Mash

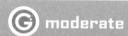 moderate

CALORIES: 187
PROTEIN: 5G
FAT: 5G
CARBOHYDRATE: 31G
FIBER: 4G

1½ lbs. sweet potatoes (about 5)

2 potatoes (about 5 ozs. each)

2 whole cloves garlic

1 tablespoon olive oil

2 sprigs fresh oregano, chopped,
or 1 tablespoon dried oregano

salt and freshly ground black pepper

1. Peel and cut the sweet potatoes and potatoes into chunks. Place in hot water in a large saucepan and add the garlic cloves.
2. Cook in plenty of salted boiling water until tender, about 20 minutes.
3. Drain and reserve ½ cup of the cooking water. Mash the drained sweet potato, potato and garlic with olive oil, chopped oregano and seasonings with a little reserved cooking water to moisten.

Serves 8 • Preparation time: 10 minutes • Cooking time: 20 minutes

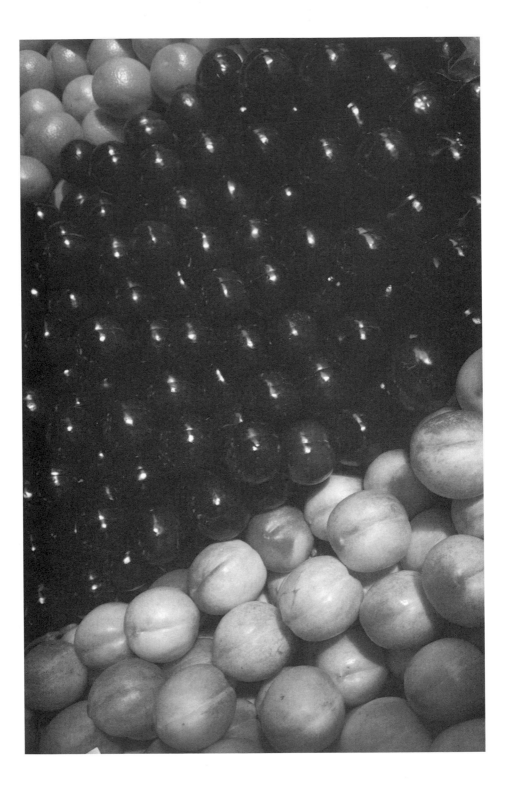

CHAPTER 14

Desserts

Mini Oat Bites

 low

CALORIES: 156
PROTEIN: 4G
FAT: 5G
CARBOHYDRATE: 27G
FIBER: 2G

3½ tablespoons margarine

2½ cups old-fashioned oats, uncooked

1 egg

½ cup sugar

1 tablespoon vanilla extract

¼ cup nonfat milk

½ cup whole wheat flour

1 teaspoon baking powder

vegetable spray

1. Preheat oven to 400°F.
2. Melt margarine in large frying pan or skillet. Add oats.
3. Cook to brown oats, about 5 minutes. Cool.
4. In large mixing bowl, beat egg and sugar until foamy. Beat in vanilla and milk.
5. Add flour and baking powder to cooled oats and mix well. Combine dry ingredients with egg mixture until well blended.
6. Using a tablespoon, scoop up the batter and with the back of another spoon, place it on a baking sheet coated with vegetable spray.
7. Bake 10 minutes. Remove form oven and allow to cool.

Makes 1½ dozen

Serves 9 • Preparation time: 20 minutes • Cooking time: 15 minutes

Poached Pears with Rich Chocolate Sauce

(G) low

CALORIES: 291
PROTEIN: 2G
FAT: 10G
CARBOHYDRATE: 54G
FIBER: 5G
OMEGA-3: *

6 medium-sized pears, peeled, cored and quartered

1 ½ quarts water

1 cup sugar

1 cinnamon stick

1 lemon (juice and zest only)

Chocolate sauce

4 ozs. dark chocolate, chopped into small pieces

1 tablespoon canola oil

5 teaspoons cold water

1. Heat the water, sugar, cinnamon stick, juice and lemon zest in a large saucepan, and simmer for 5 minutes. Add the pear slices and simmer for 20 minutes, uncovered. Cool.

2. Make the sauce by placing all the ingredients in a small saucepan. Heat gently, stirring occasionally. When combined, pour over the pears. Serve immediately with a dollop of low fat whipped cream, if desired.

Serves 6 • Preparation time: 10 minutes • Cooking time: 20 minutes

Poached Peaches in
Lemon-Ginger Syrup

 low

CALORIES: 160
PROTEIN: 2G
FAT: NEG
CARBOHYDRATE: 25G
FIBER: 2G

2 cups dry white wine

2 cups water

1 ½ teaspoons lemon zest

1 ½ tablespoons lemon juice

½" x 1" piece fresh ginger, finely sliced

½ cup sugar

6 large peaches, halved

1. Simmer the wine, water, lemon zest, lemon juice, ginger and sugar in a large saucepan for 5 minutes.
2. Add the halved peaches and poach for a further 5 minutes. Remove the peach halves with a slotted spoon and peel away their skins. Simmer the syrup to reduce by half and strain.
3. Serve peach halves with a dollop of low fat plain yogurt, and a drizzle of syrup.

Serves 6 • Preparation time: 2 minutes • Cooking time: 10 minutes

Bread and Butter Pudding

2½ cups 1% milk

4 eggs

½ cup sugar

2 teaspoons vanilla extract

2–3 slices raisin bread, crusts removed

2 teaspoons canola margarine

1. Preheat the oven to 325°F. Lightly butter a 6-cup (1½ quart) ovenproof dish.

2. Pour the milk into the dish and add the eggs, sugar and vanilla. Whisk together until combined.

3. Lightly butter the raisin bread and cut each slice diagonally. Arrange, butter side up, on top of the milk.

4. Bake for 1 hour, until the bread puffs up and turns golden brown.

Serves 4 • Preparation time: 5 minutes • Cooking time: 1 hour

Lemon Semolina Pudding
with Berry Coulis

2 cups 1% milk

½ cup fine semolina

¼ cup sugar

1 teaspoon vanilla extract

1 large lemon (zest only)

1 egg, lightly beaten

10 ozs. blackberries, strawberries, or raspberries

2 tablespoons confectioner's sugar

½ cup white wine or apple juice

1. Preheat the oven to 350°C. Lightly oil six ½-cup soufflé dishes. Line the base of each dish with baking paper.

2. Pour the milk, semolina and sugar in a saucepan and bring to a boil, stirring constantly. Reduce the heat and stir for 1 more minute.

3. Remove from the heat and stir in the vanilla extract and lemon zest.

4. Cover the surface of the mixture with plastic wrap to prevent a skin forming, and cool. When cooled, stir in the beaten egg.

5. Spoon the mixture into the prepared dishes and place them into a baking pan with enough boiling water to reach halfway up the sides of the dishes. Cover loosely with a large sheet of foil. Carefully slide the pan into the oven and poach the puddings for 15 minutes, until set. Remove the puddings from the pan of water. Run a knife around the puddings, turn out onto serving plates and remove the piece of baking paper.

6. Meanwhile, puree most of the berries with the confectioner's sugar. (Reserve some whole berries for decoration if desired). Thin the coulis with white wine or apple juice.

7. Pour the coulis around the puddings, and decorate with slivers of lemon peel or whole berries (optional).

Serves 6 • Preparation time: 10 minutes • Cooking time: 15 minutes

Individual Apple and Ginger Crumbles

Ⓖ low

CALORIES: 260
PROTEIN: 3G
FAT: 6G
CARBOHYDRATE: 50G
FIBER: 4G
OMEGA-3: *

6 Granny Smith apples, peeled, cored and sliced

1 cup water

2 tablespoons sugar

1 cinnamon stick

3 cloves

3 tablespoons glacé ginger,

coarsely chopped (optional)

Crumble

$^1/_2$ cup self-raising flour

2 tablespoons margarine

$^1/_4$ cup dark brown sugar, tightly packed

$^1/_2$ cup rolled barley

$^1/_2$ teaspoon ground nutmeg

1. Preheat the oven to 350°C. Set out six 1-cup capacity soufflé dishes.
2. Place the prepared apples, water, sugar, cinnamon stick, and cloves in a medium sized saucepan and simmer for 15 minutes, until the apples are just cooked. Remove the cinnamon stick and cloves, and mix 2 tablespoons of the glacé ginger with the apples.
3. Meanwhile, place the flour in a mixing bowl and cut the margarine through. Mix in the brown sugar, barley and nutmeg. Set aside.
4. Fill the soufflé dishes with the apples and ginger, and top with the crumble mixture.
5. Bake for 30 minutes and remove from the oven. Decorate each crumble with the remaining tablespoon of chopped ginger, and serve hot with a dollop of low fat vanilla yogurt.

Serves 6 • Preparation time: 10 minutes • Cooking time: 45 minutes

Summer Pudding

10 ozs. fresh or frozen raspberries/
blackberries/mulberries
(a few reserved for decoration)
$\frac{1}{4}$ cup raw sugar
$\frac{1}{4}$ cup red wine
$\frac{1}{4}$ cup water
1 cinnamon stick
8 slices day-old bread, crusts removed

1. Combine most of the berries, sugar, red wine, water and cinnamon stick in a medium sized saucepan and gently simmer for 5 minutes, until the berries are plump and slightly softened. Discard the cinnamon stick and cool.

2. Line a 2-cup soup bowl or mold with 6 slices of bread, cut into triangles, and overlapping so they form a casing for the berries when the pudding is turned out. Cut the remaining two slices to cover the top of the bowl.

3. Spoon a little of the berry juice over the slices to moisten them, and with a slotted spoon, fill the bowl with the berries. Pour $\frac{1}{4}$ cup of the berry juice over the berries and top with the remaining bread to make a lid. Reserve any remaining berry juice.

4. Cover with a sheet of plastic wrap, place a plate on top and weigh down with a weight. Place in the refrigerator overnight.

5. Turn out onto a white plate, decorate with reserved berries and any reserved juice, and serve with a dollop of low fat whipped cream.

Serves 4 • Preparation time: 10 minutes • Cooking time: 5 minutes

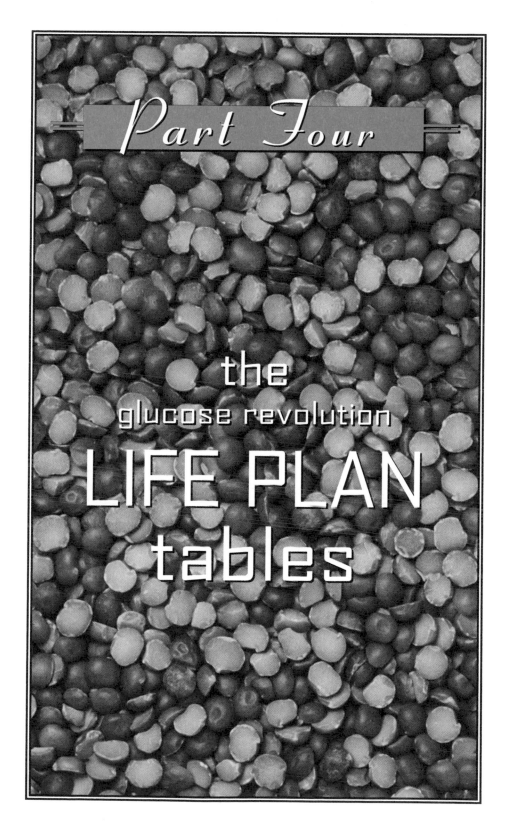

Part Four

the
glucose revolution
LIFE PLAN
tables

The Glycemic Index Tables

A-Z of Foods With Glycemic Index, Carbohydrate and Fat

The G.I. values in these tables are correct at the time of publication. However, the formulation of some commercial foods can change, which can alter the glycemic index. Check our Web page for revised and new data:

http://www.biochem.usyd.edu.au/~jennie/GI/glycemic_index.html

NOTE: You'll notice that certain foods have G.I. values exceeding 100. When measuring the glycemic index, experts use bread and glucose as the two reference foods, the standards against which the glycemic values of all other foods are measured. Glucose is used because it is the end product of digestion, and white bread is used because it is a staple in many of our diets. But foods with higher G.I. values do exist.

FOOD	GLYCEMIC INDEX	FAT (G PER SVG.)	CHO (G PER SVG.)
Agave nectar (90% fructose syrup), 1 tablespoon	11	0	12
All-Bran™, Kellogg's, breakfast cereal, ½ cup, 1 oz.	42 (av)	1	22
All-Bran with Extra Fiber™, Kellogg's, breakfast cereal, ½ cup, 1 oz.	51 (av)	1	20
Angel food cake, ¹⁄₁₂ cake, 1 oz.	67	trace	17
Apple, 1 medium, 5 ozs.	38 (av)	0	18
Apple, dried, 1 oz.	29	0	24
Apple juice, unsweetened, 1 cup, 8 ozs.	40	0	29
Apple cinnamon muffin, from mix, 1 muffin,	44	5	26
Apricots, fresh, 3 medium, 3 ozs.	57	0	12
canned, light syrup, 3 halves	64	0	14
dried, 5 halves	31	0	13
Apricot jam, no added sugar, 1 tablespoon	55	0	17
Apricot and honey muffin, low fat, from mix, 1 muffin	60	4	27
Arborio risotto rice, white, boiled, ⅔ cup	69	0	35
Bagel, 1 small, plain, 2 ozs.	72	1	38
Baked beans, ½ cup, 4 ozs.	48 (av)	1	24

FOOD	GLYCEMIC INDEX	FAT (G PER SVG.)	CHO (G PER SVG.)
Banana bread, 1 slice, 3 ozs.	47	7	46
Banana, raw, 1 medium, 5 ozs.	55 (av)	0	32
Banana, oat and honey muffin, low fat from mix, 1 muffin, small	65	4	28
Barley, pearled, boiled, 1/2 cup, 2.6 ozs.	25 (av)	0	22
Basmati white rice, boiled, 1 cup, 6 ozs.	58	0	50

Beans and legumes

FOOD	GLYCEMIC INDEX	FAT (G PER SVG.)	CHO (G PER SVG.)
Baked beans, 1/2 cup, 4 ozs.	48 (av)	1	24
Black beans, boiled, 3/4 cup, 4.3 ozs.	30	1	21
Black bean soup, 1/2 cup, 41/2 ozs.	64	2	19
Blackeyed peas, canned, 1/2 cup, 4 ozs.	42	1	16
Broad beans, canned, 1/2 cup	79	1	9
Butter beans, boiled, 1/2 cup, 4 ozs.	31 (av)	0	16
Cannellini beans	31	0	16
Chickpeas (garbanzo beans),			
canned, drained, 1/2 cup, 4 ozs.	42	2	15
boiled, 1/2 cup, 3 ozs.	33 (av)	2	23
Fava beans, frozen, boiled, 1/2 cup, 3 ozs.	79	0	17
Green pea soup, canned, ready to serve, 1 cup, 9 ozs.	66	3	27
Kidney beans, red, boiled, 1/2 cup, 3 ozs.	27 (av)	0	20
Kidney beans, red, canned and drained, 1/2 cup, 4.3 ozs.	52	0	19
Lentils, green and brown, boiled, 1/2 cup, 3 ozs.	30 (av)	0	16
Lentils, red, boiled, 1.4 cup, 4 ozs.	26 (av)	0	27
Lentil soup, Unico, canned, 1 cup, 8 ozs.	44	1	24
Lima beans, baby, frozen, 1/2 cup, 3 ozs.	32	0	17
Mung beans, boiled, 1/2 cup, 31/2 ozs.	38	1	18
Navy beans, boiled, 1/2 cup, 3 ozs.	38 (av)	0	19
Pea soup, split with ham, canned, 1 cup, 5 1/2 ozs.	66	3	25
Peas, green, fresh, frozen, boiled, 1/2 cup, 2.7 ozs.	48 (av)	0	11
Peas dried, boiled, 1/2 cup, 2 ozs.	22	0	7
Pinto beans, canned, 1/2 cup, 4 ozs.	45	1	18
Pinto beans, soaked, boiled, 1/2 cup, 3 ozs.	39	0	22
Soy beans, boiled, 1/2 cup, 3 ozs.	18 (av)	7	10
Split peas, yellow, boiled, 1/2 cup, 31/2 ozs.	32	0	21
Beets, canned, drained, 1/2 cup, 3 ozs.	64	0	5
Black bean soup, 1/2 cup, 4 1/2 ozs.	64	2	19
Black beans, boiled, 3/4 cup, 4.3 ozs.	30	1	21
Black bread, dark rye, 1 slice, 1.7 ozs.	76	1	18
Blackeyed peas, canned, 1/2 cup, 4 ozs.	42	1	16
Blueberry muffin, 1 muffin, 2 ozs.	59	4	27

FOOD	GLYCEMIC INDEX	FAT (G PER SVG.)	CHO (G PER SVG.)
Bran			
All-Bran with Extra Fiber™, Kellogg's, ½ cup, 1 oz	51	1	20
Bran Buds™,Kellogg's, ⅓ cup	58	1	14
Bran Flakes, Post, ⅔ cup, 1 oz.	74	1	22
Multi-Bran Chex™, General Mills, 1 cup, 2. ozs.	58	1.5	49
Oat bran, 1 tablespoon	55	1	7
Oat bran muffin, 2 ozs.	60	4	28
Rice bran, extruded, 1 tablespoon	19	2	3
Bran muffin, 1	60	8	34
Breads			
Dark rye, Black bread, 1 slice, 1.7 ozs.	76	1	18
Dark rye, Schinkenbröt, 1 slice, 2 ozs.	86	1	22
French baguette, 1 oz.	95	1	15
Gluten-free bread, 1 slice, 1 oz.	90	1	18
Hamburger bun, 1 prepacked bun, 1½ ozs.	61	2	22
Kaiser roll, 1, 2 ozs.	73	2	34
Light deli (American) rye, 1 slice, 1 oz.	68	1	16
Melba toast, 6 pieces, 1 oz.	70	2	23
Pita bread, whole wheat, 6½ inch loaf, 2 ozs.	57	2	35
Pumpernickel, whole grain, 1 slice, 1 oz.	51	1	16
Rye bread, 1 slice, 1 oz.	65	1	15
Sourdough, 1 slice, 1½ ozs.	52	1	20
Natural Ovens 100% Whole Grain, 1 slice, 1.2 ozs.	51	0	17
Natural Ovens Hunger Filler, 1 slice, 1.2 ozs.	59	0	16
Natural Ovens Natural Wheat, 1 slice, 1.2 ozs.	59	0	16
Natural Ovens Happiness, 1 slice, 1.1 ozs.	63	0	15
Sourdough rye, Arnold's, 1 slice, 1½ ozs.	57	1	21
White, 1 slice, 1 oz.	70 (av)	1	12
100% stoneground whole wheat, 1 slice, 1½ ozs.	53	1	12
Whole wheat, 1 slice, 1 oz.	69 (av)	1	13
Bread stuffing from mix, 2 ozs.	74	5	13
Breakfast cereals			
All-Bran™, Kellogg's, breakfast cereal, ½ cup, 1 oz.	42 (av)	1	22
All-Bran with Extra Fiber™, Kellogg's, ½ cup, 1 oz.	51	1	20
Bran Buds™,Kellogg's, ⅓ cup	58	1	14
Bran Flakes, Post, ⅔ cup, 1 oz.	74	1	22
Cheerios™, General Mills, 1 cup, 1 oz.	74	2	23
Cocoa Krispies™, Kellogg's, 1 cup, 1 oz.	77	1	27
Corn Bran™, Quaker Crunchy, ¾ cup, 1 oz.	75	1	23
Corn Chex™, Nabisco, 1 cup, 1 oz.	83	0	26

FOOD	GLYCEMIC INDEX	FAT (G PER SVG.)	CHO (G PER SVG.)
Corn Flakes™, Kellogg's, 1 cup, 1 oz.	84 (av)	0	24
Corn Pops™, 1 cup	80	0	27
Cream of Wheat, instant, 1 packet, 1 oz.	74	0	21
Cream of Wheat, old fashioned, ¾ cup, cooked, 6 ozs.	66	0	21
Crispix™, Kellogg's, 1 cup, 1 oz.	87	0	25
Frosted Flakes™, Kellogg's, ¾ cup, 1 oz.	55	0	28
Goldon Grahams™, General Mills, ¾ cup, 1.6 ozs.	71	1	25
Grapenuts™, Post, ½ cup, 1 oz.	71	1	47
Grapenuts Flakes™, Post, ¾ cup, 1 oz.	80	1	24
Just Right™, ¾ cup	60	1	36
Life™, Quaker, ¾ cup, 1 oz.	66	1	25
Mini Wheats (whole wheat), 1 cup	58	0	21
Muesli, natural muesli, ⅔ cup, 1½ ozs.	56	3	28
Muesli, breakfast cereal, toasted, ⅔ cup, 2 ozs.	43	3	41
Multi-Bran Chex™, General Mills, 1 cup, 2. ozs.	58	1.5	49
Nutri-grain™ breakfast cereal, 1 cup	66	0	20
Oat bran, raw, 1 tablespoon	55	1	7
Oat bran™, Quaker Oats, breakfast cereal, ¾ cup, 1 oz.	50	1	23
Oatmeal (made with water), old fashioned, cooked, ½ cup, 4 ozs.	49 (av)	1	12
Oats, 1-minute, Quaker Oats, 1 cup, cooked	66	2	25
Puffed Wheat™, Quaker, 2 cups, 1 oz.	80	0	22
Raisin Bran™, Kellogg's, ¾ cup, 1 oz.	73	0	32
Rice bran, 1 tablespoon	19	2	5
Rice Chex™, General Mills, 1¼ cups, 1 oz.	89	0	27
Rice Krispies™, Kellogg's, 1¼ cups, 1 oz.	82	0	26
Shredded Wheat™, Post, breakfast cereal, ½ cup, 1 oz.	83	1	23
Shredded wheat, 1 biscuit, ⅘ oz.	62	0	19
Shredded wheat, spoonsize, ⅔ cup, 1.2 ozs.	58	0	27
Smacks™, Kellogg's, ¾ cup, 1 oz.	56	1	24
Special K™, Kellogg's, 1 cup, 1 oz.	54	0	22
Team Flakes™, Nabisco, ¾ cup, 1 oz.	82	0	25
Total™, General Mills, ¾ cup, 1 oz.	76	1	27
WeetaBix™, 2 biscuits, 1.2 ozs.	75	1	28
Breton wheat crackers, 6	67	6	14
Broad beans, canned, ½ cup	79	1	9
Buckwheat groats, cooked, ½ cup, 2.7 ozs.	54 (av)	1	20
Bulgur, cooked, ⅔ cup, 4 ozs.	48 (av)	0	23
Bun, hamburger, 1 prepacked bun, 1.7 ozs.	61	2	22
Butter beans, boiled, ½ cup, 4 ozs.	31 (av)	0	16

Cakes

Angel food cake, 1 slice, 1/12 cake, 1 oz.	67	trace	17

FOOD	GLYCEMIC INDEX	FAT (G PER SVG.)	CHO (G PER SVG.)
Banana bread, 1 slice, 3 ozs.	47	7	46
Chocolate fudge cake, pkt. mix, with dark Dutch fudge frosting, Betty Crocker, 1/12 of cake, with 2 tablespoons frosting	38	17	54
French vanilla cake, pkt. mix, with vanilla frosting, Betty Crocker, 1/12 of cake, with 2 tablespoons frosting	42	15	58
Pound cake, homemade, 1 slice, 3 ozs.	54	15	42
Sponge cake, 1 slice, 1/12 cake, 2 ozs.	46	4	32
Capellini pasta, cooked, 1 cup, 6 ozs.	45	1	53
Cannellini beans, boiled, 1/2 cup, 4 ozs.	31	0	16
Cantaloupe, raw, 1/4 small, 6 1/2 ozs.	65	0	16
Carrots, peeled, boiled, 1/2 cup, 2.4 ozs.	49	0	3

Cereal grains

FOOD	GLYCEMIC INDEX	FAT (G PER SVG.)	CHO (G PER SVG.)
Barley, pearled, boiled, 1/2 cup, 2.6 ozs.	25 (av)	0	22
Bulgur, cooked, 1/2 cup, 3 ozs.	48 (av)	0	17
Couscous, cooked, 1/2 cup, 3 ozs.	65 (av)	0	21
Corn			
Cornmeal, whole grain, from mix, cooked, 1/3 cup, 1.4 ozs.	68	1	30
Corn, canned, drained, 1/2 cup, 3 ozs.	55 (av)	1	15
Taco shells, 2 shells, 1 oz.	68	5	17
Rice			
Basmati, white, boiled, 1 cup, 6 ozs.	58	0	50
Brown, 1 cup, 6 ozs.	55 (av)	0	37
Converted™, Uncle Ben's, 1 cup, 6 ozs.	44	38	
Instant, cooked, 1 cup, 6 ozs.	87	0	37
Long grain, white, 1 cup, 6 ozs.	56 (av)	0	42
Parboiled, 1 cup, 6 ozs.	48	0	38
Rice cakes, plain, 3 cakes, 1 oz.	82	1	23
Short grain, white, 1 cup, 6 ozs.	72	0	42
Chana dal, 1/2 cup, 4 ozs.	8	3	28
Cheerios™, General Mills, breakfast cereal, 1 cup, 1 oz.	74	2	23
Cherries, 10 large cherries, 3 ozs.	22	0	10
Chickpeas (garbanzo beans),			
canned, drained, 1/2 cup, 4 ozs.	42	2	15
boiled, 1/2 cup, 3 ozs.	33 (av)	2	23
Chocolate butterscotch muffin, low fat from mix, 1 muffin	53	4	28
Chocolate, bar, 1 1/2 ozs.	49	14	26
Chocolate Flavor, Nestle Quik™ (made with water), 3 teaspoons	53	0	14
Chocolate fudge cake, pkt. mix, with dark Dutch fudge frosting, Betty Crocker, 1/12 of cake, with 2 tablespoons frosting	38	17	54
Coca-Cola™, soft drink, 1 can	63	0	41
Cocoa Krispies™, Kellogg's, breakfast cereal, 1 cup, 1 oz.	77	1	27

FOOD	GLYCEMIC INDEX	FAT (G PER SVG.)	CHO (G PER SVG.)
Corn			
Cornmeal (polenta), 1/3 cup, 1.4 ozs.	68	1	30
Corn, canned and drained, 1/2 cup, 3 ozs.	55 (av)	1	15
Corn Bran™, Quaker Crunchy, breakfast cereal, 3/4 cup, 1 oz.	75	1	23
Corn Chex™, General Mills, breakfast cereal, 1 cup, 1 oz.	83	0	
Corn chips, 1 oz.	72	10	16
Corn Flakes™, Kellogg's, breakfast cereal, 1 cup, 1 oz.	84 (av)	0	24
Corn Pops™, 1 cup	80	0	27
Cornmeal, from mix, cooked, 1/3 cup, 1.4 ozs.	68	1	30
Cookies			
Graham crackers, 4 squares, 1 oz.	74	3	22
Milk Arrowroot, 3 cookies, 1/2 oz.	69	2	9
Oatmeal, 1 cookie, 2/3 oz.	55	3	12
Shortbread, 4 small cookies, 1 oz.	64	7	19
Social Tea™ biscuits, Nabisco, 4 cookies, 2/3 oz.	55	3	13
Vanilla wafers, 7 cookies, 1 oz.	77	4	21
see also Crackers			
Couscous, cooked, 2/3 cup, 4 ozs.	65 (av)	0	21
Crackers			
Breton wheat crackers, 6	67	6	14
Crispbread, 3 crackers, 2/3 oz.	81	0	15
Kavli™ All Natural Whole Grain Crispbread, 4 wafers, 1 oz.	71	1	16
Premium saltine crackers, 8 crackers, 1 oz.	74	3	17
Rice cakes, plain, 3 cakes, 1 oz.	82	1	23
Ryvita™ Tasty Dark Rye Whole Grain Crisp Bread, 2 slices, 2/3 oz.	69	1	16
Stoned wheat thins, 3 crackers, 4/5 oz.	67	2	15
Water cracker, Carr's, 3 king size crackers, 4/5 oz.	78	2	18
Cranberry juice cocktail, 8 ozs.	52	0	31
Cream of Wheat, instant, 1 packet, 1 oz.	74	0	21
Cream of Wheat, old fashioned, 3/4 cup, cooked, 6 ozs.	66	0	21
Crispix™, Kellogg's, breakfast cereal, 1 cup, 1 oz.	87	0	25
Croissant, medium, 1.2 ozs.	67	14	27
Cupcake, with icing and cream filling, 1 cake	73	3	26
Custard, 3/4 cup, 4.4 ozs.	43	5	36
Dairy foods and nondairy substitutes			
Ice cream, 10% fat, vanilla, 1/2 cup, 2.2 ozs.	61 (av)	7	16
Ice milk, vanilla, 1/2 cup, 2.2 ozs.	50	3	15
Milk, whole, 1 cup, 8 ozs.	27 (av)	9	11
skim, 1 cup, 8 ozs.	32	0	12
chocolate flavored, 1%, 1 cup, 8 ozs.	34	3	26

FOOD	GLYCEMIC INDEX	FAT (G PER SVG.)	CHO (G PER SVG.)
Pudding, ½ cup, 4.4 ozs.	43	4	27
Soy milk, 1 cup, 8 ozs.	31	7	14
Tofu frozen dessert (nondairy), low fat, ½ cup, 2 ozs.	115	1	21
Yogurt			
nonfat, fruit flavored, with sugar, 8 ozs.	33	0	30
nonfat, plain, artificial sweetener, 8 ozs.	14	0	17
nonfat, fruit flavored, artificial sweetener, 8 ozs.	14	0	17
Dates, dried, 5, 1.4 ozs.	103	0	27
Doughnut with cinnamon and sugar, 1.6 ozs.	76	11	29
Fanta™, soft drink, 1 can	68	0	47
Fava beans, frozen, boiled, ½ cup, 3 ozs.	79	0	17
Fettucine, cooked, 1 cup, 6 ozs.	32	1	57
Fish sticks, frozen, oven-cooked, fingers, 3½ sticks	38	14	24
Flan (creme caramel), ½ cup, 4 ozs.	65	5	23
French baguette bread, 1 oz., about one 1-inch slice	95	0	15
French fries, large, 4.3 ozs.	75	22	46
French vanilla cake, pkt. mix, with vanilla frosting, Betty Crocker, ¹⁄₁₂ of cake, with 2 tablespoons frosting	42	15	58
Frosted Flakes™, Kellogg's, breakfast cereal, ¾ cup, 1 oz.	55	0	28
Fructose, pure, 3 packets	23 (av)	0	10
Fruit cocktail, canned in natural juice, ½ cup, 4 ozs.	55	0	15

Fruits and fruit products

FOOD	GLYCEMIC INDEX	FAT (G PER SVG.)	CHO (G PER SVG.)
Agave nectar (90% fructose syrup), 1 tablespoon	11	0	12
Apple, 1 medium, 5 ozs.	38 (av)	0	18
Apple, dried, 1 oz.	29	0	24
Apple juice, unsweetened, 1 cup, 8 ozs.	40	0	29
Apricots, fresh, 3 medium, 3.3 ozs.	57	0	12
canned, light syrup, 3 halves	64	0	19
dried, 1 oz.	31	0	13
Apricot jam, no added sugar, 1 tablespoon	55	0	17
Banana, raw, 1 medium, 5 ozs.	55 (av)	0	32
Cherries, 10 large, 3 ozs.	22	0	10
Cranberry juice cocktail, 8 ozs.	52	0	31
Dates, dried, 5, 1.4 ozs.	103	0	27
Fruit cocktail, canned in natural juice, ½ cup, 4 ozs.	55	0	15
Grapefruit, raw, ½ medium, 3.3 ozs.	25	0	5
Grapefruit juice, unsweetened, 1 cup, 8 ozs.	48	0	22
Grapes, green, 1 cup, 3 ozs.	46 (av)	0	15
Kiwi, 1 medium, raw, peeled, 2½ ozs.	52 (av)	0	8
Lychee, canned and drained, 7	79	0	16
Mango, 1 small, 5 ozs.	55 (av)	0	19

FOOD	GLYCEMIC INDEX	FAT (G PER SVG.)	CHO (G PER SVG.)
Marmalade, 1 tablespoon	48	0	17
Orange, navel, 1 medium, 4 ozs.	44 (av)	0	10
Orange juice, 1 cup, 8 ozs.	46	0	26
Papaya, 1/2 medium, 5 ozs.	58 (av)	0	14
Peach, fresh, 1 medium, 3 ozs.	30	0	7
canned, natural juice, 1/2 cup, 4 ozs.	30	0	14
canned, light syrup, 1/2 cup, 4 ozs.	52	0	18
canned, heavy syrup, 1/2 cup, 4 ozs.	58	0	26
Pear, fresh, 1 medium, 5 ozs.	38 (av)	0	21
canned in pear juice, 1/2 cup, 4 ozs.	44	0	13
Pineapple, fresh, 2 slices, 4 ozs.	66	0	10
Pineapple juice, unsweetened, canned, 8 ozs.	46	0	34
Plums, 1 medium, 2 ozs.	39 (av)	0	7
Prunes, pitted, 6	29	0	25
Raisins, 1/4 cup, 1 oz.	64	0	28
Strawberry jam, 1 tablespoon	51	0	18
Watermelon, 1 cup, 5 ozs.	72	0	8
Gatorade™ sports drink, 1 cup, 8 ozs.	78	0	14
Glucose powder, 2 1/2 tablets	102	0	10
Gluten-free bread, 1 slice, 1 oz.	90	1	18
Glutinous rice, white, steamed, 1 cup	98	0	37
Gnocchi, cooked, 1 cup, 5 ozs.	68	3	71
Golden Grahams™, General Mills, 3/4 cup, 1.6 ozs.	71	1	25
Graham crackers, 4 squares, 1 oz.	74	3	22
Granola Bars™, Quaker Chewy, 1 oz.	61	2	23
Grapefruit, raw, 1/2 medium, 3.3 ozs.	25	0	5
Grapefruit juice unsweetened, 1 cup, 8 ozs.	48	0	22
Grapenuts™, Post, breakfast cereal, 1/2 cup, 1 oz.	71	1	47
Grapenuts Flakes™, Post, breakfast cereal, 3/4 cup, 1 oz.	80	1	24
Grapes, green, 1 cup, 3.3 ozs.	46 (av)	0	15
Green pea soup, canned, ready to serve, 1 cup, 9 ozs.	66	3	27
Hamburger bun, 1 prepacked bun, 1 1/2 ozs.	61	2	22
Honey, 1 tablespoon	58	0	16
Ice cream, 10% fat, vanilla, 1/2 cup, 2.2 ozs.	61 (av)	7	16
Ice milk, vanilla, 1/2 cup, 2.2 ozs.	50	3	15
Isostar, 1 cup, 8 ozs.	70	0	18
Jasmine, white, long grain, steamed, 1 cup	109	0	39
Jelly beans, 10 large, 1 oz.	80	0	26
Just Right™, breakfast cereal, 3/4 cup	60	1	36
Kaiser rolls, 1 roll, 2 ozs.	73	2	34
Kavli™ All Natural Whole Grain Crispbread, 4 wafers, 1 oz.	71	1	16

FOOD	GLYCEMIC INDEX	FAT (G PER SVG.)	CHO (G PER SVG.)
Kidney beans, red, boiled, 1/2 cup, 3 ozs.	27 (av)	0	20
Kidney beans, red, canned and drained, 1/2 cup, 4.3 ozs.	52	0	19
Kiwi, 1 medium, raw, peeled, 2 1/2 ozs.	52 (av)	0	8
Kudos Granola Bars™ (whole grain), 1 bar, 1 oz.	62	5	20
Lactose, pure, 7/10 oz.	46 (av)	0	10
Lentil soup, Unico, canned, 1 cup, 8 ozs.	44	1	24
Lentils, green and brown, boiled, 1/2 cup, 3 ozs.	30 (av)	0	16
Lentils, red, boiled, 1.4 cup, 4 ozs.	26 (av)	0	27
Life™, Quaker, breakfast cereal, 3/4 cup, 1 oz.	66	1	25
Life Savers™, roll candy, 6 pieces, peppermint	70	0	10
Light deli (American) rye bread, 1 slice, 1 oz.	68	1	16
Lima beans, baby, frozen, 1/2 cup, 3 ozs.	32	0	17
Linguine pasta, thick, cooked, 1 cup, 6 ozs.	46 (av)	1	56
Linguine pasta, thin, cooked, 1 cup, 6 ozs.	55 (av)	1	56
Lychee, canned and drained, 7	79	0	16
M&M's Chocolate Candies Peanut™, 1.7 oz. package	33	13	30
Macaroni and Cheese Dinner™, Kraft packaged, cooked, 1 cup, 7 ozs.	64	17	48
Macaroni, cooked, 1 cup, 6 ozs.	45	1	42
Maltose (maltodextrin), pure, 2 1/2 teaspoons	105	0	10
Mango, 1 small, 5 ozs.	55 (av)	0	19
Marmalade, 1 tablespoon	48	0	17
Mars Almond Bar™, 1.8 ozs.	65	12	31
Mars Bar™, 1 bar	65	11	41
Melba toast, 6 pieces, 1 oz.	70	1	23
Milk, whole, 1 cup, 8 ozs.	27 (av)	9	11
skim, 1 cup, 8 ozs.	32	0	12
chocolate flavored, 1%, 1 cup, 8 ozs.	34	3	26
Milk Arrowroot, 3 cookies, 1/2 oz.	63	2	9
Millet, cooked, 1/2 cup, 4 ozs.	71	1	28
Mini Wheats (whole wheat), breakfast cereal, 1 cup	58	0	21
Muesli, breakfast cereal, toasted, 2/3 cup, 2 ozs.	43	3	41
Muesli, non-toasted, 2/3 cup, 1 1/2 ozs.	56	3	28
Multi-Bran Chex™, General Mills, 1 cup, 2. ozs.	58	1.5	49
Muffins			
Apple cinnamon, from mix, 1 muffin, 2 ozs.	44	8	33
Apricot and honey, low fat, from mix, 1 muffin	60	4	27
Banana, oat and honey, low fat, from mix, 1 muffin, small	65	4	28
Blueberry, 1 muffin, 2 ozs.	59	4	27
Bran, 1 muffin	60	8	34
Chocolate butterscotch, low fat, from mix, 1 muffin	53	4	28

FOOD	GLYCEMIC INDEX	FAT (G PER SVG.)	CHO (G PER SVG.)
Oat and raisin, low fat, from mix, 1 muffin	54	3	28
Oat bran, 1 muffin, 2 ozs.	60	4	28
Mung beans, boiled, 1/2 cup, 31/2 ozs.	38	1	18
Mung bean noodles, 1 cup	39	0	35
Natural Ovens 100% Whole Grain bread, 1 slice, 1.2 ozs.	51	0	17
Natural Ovens Hunger Filler bread, 1 slice, 1.2 ozs.	59	0	16
Natural Ovens Natural Wheat bread, 1 slice, 1.2 ozs.	59	0	16
Natural Ovens Happiness bread, 1 slice, 1.1 ozs.	63	0	15
Navy beans, boiled, 1/2 cup, 3 ozs.	38 (av)	0	19
Noodles, mung bean, 1 cup	39	0	35
Nutella™ (spread), 2 tablespoons	33	9	19
Nutri-grain™ breakfast cereal, 1 cup	66	0	20
Oat and raisin muffin, low fat from mix, 1 muffin	54	3	28
Oat bran, 1 tablespoon	55	1	7
Oat bran™, Quaker Oats, breakfast cereal, 3/4 cup, 1 oz.	50	1	23
Oat bran, 1 muffin, 2 ozs.	60	4	28
Oatmeal (made with water), old fashioned, cooked, 1/2 cup, 4 ozs.	49	1	12
Oatmeal cookie, 1, 2/5 oz.	55	3	12
Oats, 1-minute, Quaker Oats, 1 cup, cooked	66	2	25
Orange, navel, 1 medium, 4 ozs.	44 (av)	0	10
Orange syrup, diluted, 1 cup	66	0	20
Orange juice, 1 cup, 8 ozs.	46	0	26
Papaya, 1/2 medium, 5 ozs.	58 (av)	0	14
Parsnips, boiled, 1/2 cup, 21/2 ozs.	97	0	15

Pasta

FOOD	GLYCEMIC INDEX	FAT (G PER SVG.)	CHO (G PER SVG.)
Capellini, cooked, 1 cup, 6 ozs.	45	1	53
Fettuccine, cooked, 1 cup, 6 ozs.	32	1	57
Gnocchi, cooked, 1 cup, 5 ozs.	68	3	71
Linguine thick, cooked, 1 cup, 6 ozs.	46 (av)	1	56
Linguine thin, cooked, 1 cup, 6 ozs.	55 (av)	1	56
Macaroni, cooked, 1 cup, 5 ozs.	45	1	42
Macaroni & Cheese Dinner™, Kraft, packaged, cooked, 1 cup, 7 ozs.	64	17	48
Ravioli, meat-filled, cooked, 4 large	39	6	41
Spaghetti, white, cooked, 1 cup, 6 ozs.	41 (av)	1	42
Spaghetti, whole wheat, cooked, 1 cup, 6 ozs.	37 (av)	1	48
Spirali, durum, cooked, 1 cup, 6 ozs.	43	1	56
Star Pastina, cooked, 1 cup, 6 ozs.	38	1	56
Tortellini, cheese, cooked, 8 ozs.	50	7	28
Vermicelli, cooked, 1 cup, 6 ozs.	35	0	42
Pastry, flaky, 1/8 of double crust, 2 ozs.	59	15	24

FOOD	GLYCEMIC INDEX	FAT (G PER SVG.)	CHO (G PER SVG.)
Pea soup, split with ham, canned, 1 cup, 5½ ozs.	66	3	25
Peach, fresh, 1 medium, 3 ozs.	30	0	7
canned, heavy syrup, ½ cup, 4 ozs.	58	0	26
canned, light syrup, ½ cup, 4 ozs.	52	0	18
canned, natural juice, ½ cup, 4 ozs.	30	0	14
Peanuts, roasted, salted, ½ cup, 1.1 oz. bag	15 (av)	38	7
Pear, fresh, 1 medium, 5 ozs.	38 (av)	0	21
canned in pear juice, ½ cup, 4 ozs.	44	0	13
Peas, green, fresh, frozen, boiled, ½ cup, 2.7 ozs.	48 (av)	0	10
Peas, dried, boiled, ½ cup, 2 ozs.	22	0	12
Pineapple, fresh, 2 slices, 4 ozs.	66	0	10
Pineapple juice, unsweetened, canned, 8 ozs.	46	0	34
Pinto beans, canned, ½ cup, 4 ozs.	45	1	18
Pinto beans, soaked, boiled, ½ cup, 3 ozs.	39	0	22
Pita bread, whole wheat, 6½ inch loaf, 2 ozs.	57	2	35
Pizza, cheese and tomato, 2 slices, 8 ozs.	60	22	56
Pizza, Super Supreme, Pizza Hut, pan, 2 slices	36	31	72
Pizza, Super Supreme, Pizza Hut, thin and crispy, 2 slices	30	27	50
Plums, 1 medium, 2 ozs.	39 (av)	0	7
Popcorn, light, microwave, 1¾ oz. snack size	55	8	30
Pop Tarts™, double chocolate, 1 tart	70	5	36
Potatoes			
Desirée, peeled, boiled, 1 medium, 4 ozs.	101	0	13
French fries, large, 4.3 ozs.	75	26	49
instant mashed potatoes, Carnation Foods™, ½ cup, 3½ ozs.	86	2	14
new, unpeeled, boiled, 4 medium, 6 ozs.	78 (av)	0	25
new, canned, drained, 5 small, 6 ozs.	61	0	26
red-skinned, peeled, boiled, 1 medium, 4 ozs.	88 (av)	0	15
red-skinned, baked in oven (no fat), 1 medium, 4 ozs.	93 (av)	0	15
red-skinned, mashed, ½ cup, 4 ozs.	91 (av)	0	16
red-skinned, microwaved, 1 medium, 4 ozs.	79	0	15
sweet potato, peeled, boiled, mashed, ½ cup, 3 ozs.	54 (av)	0	20
white-skinned, peeled, boiled, 1 medium, 4 ozs.	63 (av)	0	24
white-skinned, with skin, baked in oven (no fat), 1 medium, 4 ozs.	85 (av)	0	30
white-skinned, mashed, ½ cup, 4 ozs.	70 (av)	0	20
white-skinned, with skin, microwaved, 1 medium, 4 ozs.	82	0	29
Sebago, peeled, boiled, 1 medium, 4 ozs.	87	0	13
Potato chips, plain, 14 pieces, 1 oz.	54 (av)	10	15
Pound cake, 1 slice, homemade, 3 ozs.	54	15	42

FOOD	GLYCEMIC INDEX	FAT (G PER SVG.)	CHO (G PER SVG.)
Power Bar™, Performance, Chocolate, 1 bar	58	2	45
Premium saltine crackers, 8 crackers, 1 oz.	74	3	17
Pretzels, 1 oz.	83	1	22
Prunes, pitted, 6	29	0	25
Puffed Wheat™, Quaker, breakfast cereal, 2 cups, 1 oz.	80	0	22
Pumpernickel bread, whole grain, 2 slices	51	2	32
Pumpkin, peeled, boiled, mashed, 1/2 cup, 4 ozs.	75	0	6
Raisins, 1/4 cup, 1 oz.	64	0	28
Raisin Bran™, Kellogg's, breakfast cereal, 3/4 cup, 1.3 ozs.	73	0	32
Ravioli, meat-filled, cooked, 1 cup, 4 large	39	6	41

Rice

FOOD	GLYCEMIC INDEX	FAT (G PER SVG.)	CHO (G PER SVG.)
Arborio risotto rice, white, boiled, 2/3 cup	69	0	35
Basmati, white, boiled, 1 cup, 7 ozs.	58	0	50
Brown, 1 cup, 6 ozs.	55 (av)	0	37
Converted™, Uncle Ben's, 1 cup, 6 ozs.	44	0	38
Glutinous, white, steamed, 1 cup	98	0	37
Instant, cooked, 1 cup, 6 ozs.	87	0	38
Jasmine, white, long grain, steamed, 1 cup	109	0	39
Long grain, white, 1 cup, 6 ozs.	56 (av)	0	42
Parboiled, 1 cup, 6 ozs.	48	0	38
Rice bran, extruded, 1 tablespoon	19	2	3
Rice cakes, plain, 3 cakes, 1 oz.	82	1	23
Short grain, white, 1 cup, 6 ozs.	72	0	42
Rice Chex™, General Mills, breakfast cereal, 1 1/4 cups, 1 oz.	89	0	27
Rice Krispies™, Kellogg's, breakfast cereal, 1 1/4 cups, 1 oz.	82	0	26
Rice vermicelli, cooked, 6 ozs.	58	0	48
Roll (bread), Kaiser, 1 roll, 2 ozs.	73	2	39
Roll-ups™, 1 fruit leather	99	1	13
Romano (cranberry) beans, boiled, 1/2 cup, 3 ozs.	46	0	21
Rutabaga, peeled, boiled, 1/2 cup, 2.6 ozs.	72	0	3
Rye bread, 1 slice, 1 oz.	65	1	15
Ryvita™ Tasty Dark Rye Whole Grain Crisp Bread, 2 slices, 2/3 oz.	69	1	16
Semolina, cooked, 1 cup, 6 ozs.	55	0	17
Shortbread, 4 small cookies, 1 oz.	64	7	19
Shredded Wheat™, Post, breakfast cereal, 1 oz.	83	1	23
Shredded wheat, 1 biscuit, 4/5 oz.	62	0	19
Shredded wheat, spoonsize, 2/3 cup, 1.2 ozs.	58	0	27
Skittles Original Fruit Bite Size Candies™, 2.3 oz. pk.	70	3	59
Smacks™, Kellogg's, breakfast cereal, 3/4 cup, 1 oz.	56	1	27
Snickers™, 2.2 oz. bar	41	15	36
Social Tea™ biscuits, Nabisco, 4 cookies, 2/3 oz.	55	3	13

FOOD	GLYCEMIC INDEX	FAT (G PER SVG.)	CHO (G PER SVG.)
Soft drink, Coca-Cola™, 1 can, 12 ozs.	63	0	39
Soft drink, Fanta™, 1 can, 12 ozs.	68	0	47
Soups			
Black bean soup, ½ cup, 4½ ozs.	64	2	19
Green pea soup, canned, ready to serve, 1 cup, 9 ozs.	66	3	27
Lentil soup, Unico, canned, 1 cup, 8 ozs.	44	1	24
Pea soup, split with ham, 1 cup, 5½ ozs.	66	3	25
Tomato soup, canned, 1 cup, 9 ozs.	38	4	36
Sourdough bread, 1 slice, 1½ ozs.	52	1	20
Rye bread, Arnold's, 1 slice, 1½ ozs.	57	1	21
Soy beans, boiled, ½ cup, 3 ozs.	18 (av)	7	10
Soy milk, 1 cup, 8 ozs.	31	7	14
Spaghetti, white, cooked, 1 cup	41 (av)	1	42
Spaghetti, whole wheat, cooked, 1 cup, 5 ozs.	37 (av)	1	48
Special K™, Kellogg's, breakfast cereal, 1 cup, 1 oz.	54	0	22
Spirali, durum, cooked, 1 cup, 6 ozs.	43	1	56
Split pea soup, 8 ozs.	60	4	38
Split peas, yellow, boiled, ½ cup, 3½ ozs.	32	0	29
Sponge cake plain, 1 slice, 3½ ozs.	46	4	32
Sports drinks			
Gatorade™ 1 cup, 8 ozs.	78	0	14
Isostar, 1 cup, 8 ozs.	70	0	18
Sportsplus, 1 cup, 8 ozs.	74	0	17
Power Bar™, Performance Chocolate Bar, 1 bar	58	3	45
Stoned wheat thins, 3 crackers, ⅘ oz.	67	2	15
Strawberry Nestle Quik™ (made with water), 3 teaspoons	64	0	14
Strawberry jam, 1 tablespoon	51	0	18
Sucrose, 1 teaspoon	65 (av)	0	4
Super Supreme pizza, Pizza Hut, pan, 2 slices	36	31	72
Super Supreme pizza, Pizza Hut, thin and crispy, 2 slices	30	27	50
Syrup, fruit flavored, diluted, 1 cup	66	0	20
Sweet potato, peeled, boiled, mashed, ½ cup, 3 ozs.	54 (av)	0	20
Taco shells, 2 shells, 1 oz.	68	5	17
Tapioca pudding, boiled with whole milk, 1 cup, 10 ozs.	81	13	51
Taro, peeled, boiled, ½ cup, 2 ozs.	54	0	23
Team Flakes™, Nabisco, breakfast cereal, ¾ cup, 1 oz.	82	0	25
Tofu frozen dessert, nondairy, low fat, 2 ozs.	115	1	21
Tomato soup, canned, 1 cup, 9 ozs.	38	4	33
Tortellini, cheese, cooked, 8 ozs.	50	7	28

FOOD	GLYCEMIC INDEX	FAT (G PER SVG.)	CHO (G PER SVG.)
Total™, General Mills, breakfast cereal, ¾ cup, 1 oz.	76	1	24
Twix Chocolate Caramel Cookie™, 2, 2 ozs.	44	14	37
Vanilla wafers, 7 cookies, 1 oz.	77	4	21
Vermicelli, cooked, 1 cup, 6 ozs.	35	0	42
Vitasoy™ Soy milk, creamy original, 1 cup, 8 ozs.	31	7	14
Waffles, plain, frozen, 4 inch square, 1 oz.	76	3	13
Water crackers, 3 king size crackers, ⅘ oz.	78	2	18
Watermelon, 1 cup, 5 ozs	72	0	8
Weetabix™ breakfast cereal, 2 biscuits, 1.2 ozs.	75	1	28
White bread, 1 slice, 1 oz.	70 (av)	1	12
Whole wheat bread, 1 slice, 1 oz.	69 (av)	1	13
Yam, boiled, 3 ozs.	51	0	24

Yogurt

FOOD	GLYCEMIC INDEX	FAT (G PER SVG.)	CHO (G PER SVG.)
nonfat, fruit flavored, with sugar, 8 ozs.	33	0	30
nonfat, plain, artificial sweetener, 8 ozs.	14	0	17
nonfat, fruit flavored, artificial sweetener, 8 ozs.	14	0	17

Alpha-linolenic acid (ALA): The plant form of polyunsaturated omega-3 fat. ALA is found in linseed, canola, walnut and soybean oils. There are also small amounts in walnuts, linseeds, pecans, soybeans, baked beans, wheat germ, lean meats, and green leafy vegetables.

Antioxidant: Any substance that inhibits the oxidation of another substance. Oxidation is a natural process that occurs in our bodies all the time, but it is implicated specifically in such conditions as cardiovascular disease, cancer and aging. Dietary antioxidants, such as vitamins C and E, are believed to limit these disease processes.

Asian diet: A low-fat diet consisting primarily of seafood, rice and varying amounts of vegetables and fruits. People eating this diet tend to have lower rates of heart disease, type 2 diabetes and cancer.

Atherosclerosis: Also known as hardening of the arteries, this condition can lead to heart disease.

Carbohydrates: Carbohydrates are our bodies' preferred fuel source. They consist of glucose, in addition to one or more other compounds containing carbon, hydrogen and oxygen atoms. Because of their chemical composition, it is easiest for our bodies to break down carbohydrate foods into energy.

Carotenoids: These phytochemicals are heart-healthy and help prevent certain cancers. Carotenoids are found in yellow and orange fruits and vegetables, as well as in dark green leafy vegetables.

Cytokine: A blood substance that initiates our body's immune response and its consequent inflammation. Scientists believe that omega-3 fatty acids decrease these reactions.

Daidzein: An isoflavone in soy that may lower the risk of some forms of cancer.

DASH diet: This study (**D**ietary **A**pproaches to **S**top **H**ypertension) found that very high fruit, vegetable and nut intakes reduced blood pressure. The results in mildly hypertensive patients far exceeded the results of other non-drug treatments (such as low-salt diets) and are similar to results from drug therapy.

Docosahexanoic Acid (DHA): This essential fatty acid helps to control high blood pressure and is associated with lower risks of rheumatoid arthritis, depression and cancer. Fatty fish, such as shellfish, mackerel, tuna, salmon, bluefish, mullet, sturgeon, anchovy, herring, trout, sardines are all good food sources.

Eicosanoid: A substance in the blood that initiates our body's immune response and the resulting inflammation. Scientists believe that omega-3 fatty acids decrease these reactions.

Eicosapentanoic Acid (EPA): This essential fatty acid helps to control high blood pressure and is associated with lower risks of rheumatoid arthritis, depression and cancer. Fatty fish, such as shellfish, mackerel, tuna, salmon, bluefish, mullet, sturgeon, anchovy, herring, trout, sardines are all good food sources.

Flavonoids: These phytochemicals with antioxidant properties help to prevent tumor formation. Flavonoids are especially prevalent in soy foods,

Genistein: An estrogen-like substance, or isoflavone, found in soy beans, which has been proven to lower the risk of some forms of cancer.

Glycemic index: A numerical ranking of foods based on their immediate effect on our blood sugar levels. Carbohydrate foods that break down quickly during digestion have the highest G.I. values because the blood sugar response is fast and high. Carbohydrates that break down slowly, releasing glucose gradually into the bloodstream, have low G.I. values.

HDL cholesterol: High-density lipoprotein cholesterol, also known as "good" cholesterol because elevated levels of this blood fat protect against heart disease.

High G.I. food: A food with a glycemic index greater than 70. High G.I. foods raise blood sugar levels the most.

Homocysteine: A substance normally produced when our bodies metabolize the amino acid methionine. Elevated levels of homocysteine are associated with an increased risk of heart disease.

Indoles: Found in cruciferous vegetables such as broccoli, cauliflower, cabbage and Brussels sprouts, this phytochemical may reduce breast cancer risk.

Insulin: A hormone produced by the pancreas, which helps to metabolize carbohydrates and is used to manage and treat diabetes.

Isoflavones: A type of phytoestrogen (the plant form of estrogen) found in soybeans.

LDL cholesterol: Low-density lipoprotein cholesterol, also known as "bad" cholesterol. Elevated levels of this type of blood fat are a risk factor for heart disease.

Lipids: Another term for fats. Cholesterol and triglycerides are all blood lipids.

Low G.I. food: A food with a glycemic index less than 55. Low G.I. foods raise blood sugar levels least.

Lycopene: This chemical gives tomatoes and pink grapefruit their red pigment, and has strong anti-cancer and antioxidant properties.

Macronutrients: The major nutrients that our bodies require, including protein, fat, carbohydrate and water.

Mediterranean diet: A diet consisting primarily of fish, fruits, vegetables, olives and olive oil. People eating this diet tend to have lower rates of heart disease and cancer.

Metabolism: The process by which our bodies use nutrients for energy and to dispose of waste products.

Micronutrients: Nutrients that are present in foods and that our bodies require in relatively small amounts, including vitamins and minerals.

Monounsaturated fats (MUFAs): Oleic acid is one example of a MUFA. These heart-healthy fats are liquid at room temperature.

Nitrosamines: Potentially cancer-causing substances formed by amines and nitrites in foods.

Omega-3 (Linolenic Acid): Omega-3 is an essential fatty acid that our bodies cannot produce. Studies show that this fatty acid can reduce arthritis pain and cancer risk and aid in brain development. Good food sources include fats and oils (canola, soybean, walnut, wheat germ and some margarines), nuts and seeds (butternuts, walnuts, soybean kernels) and soybeans.

Omega-6 (Linoleic Acid): Our bodies can't make linoleic acid, so we must get it from the foods we eat. Omega-6 fatty acids aid in cell membrane integrity, blood pressure regulation, blood clot formation, regulation of blood lipids and immune response to injury and infection. Good food sources include leafy vegetables, seeds, nuts, grains, vegetable oils, including corn, safflower, soybean, cottonseed, sesame and sunflower.

Paleolithic diet: A high-fiber diet that probably consisted of 65 percent animal food and 35 percent plant foods, including fruit, roots, legumes and nuts. Experts speculate that this high-fiber diet would have lowered the incidence of diabetes, colon cancer and anemia.

Phytochemicals: Natural chemicals, found in all plant foods, that can be beneficial to health.

Phytoestrogens: Plant chemicals that are similar in structure to the estrogens our bodies produce and that have similar, although weaker, effects. Examples include isoflavones in soy and lignins in linseed.

Polyphenols: A group of phytochemicals found in fruits, grains, vegetables, wine, tea, cocoa and chocolate, which is believed to have antioxidant properties.

Polyunsaturated fats (PUFAs): Liquid at room temperature, examples of PUFAs include linoleic acid and linolenic acid. PUFAs are found in all vegetable oils, especially safflower, sunflower, corn, soybean and cottonseed.

Saturated fat: Solid at room temperature (such as butter, for example), saturated fat comes in the form of fatty marbling in meat, the cream in milk and other high fat dairy products, and in some of the tropical oils such as palm oil, widely used as shortening for frying and for making cakes, pies, cookies and crackers. Studies show that saturated fat increases our risk of heart disease, obesity and certain cancers.

Selenium: A mineral often grouped with antioxidants; it may help to prevent cancer.

Squalene: An antioxidant substance found in olive oil.

Sugar: There are six common sugars found in foods: glucose (in all fruits and some vegetables); fructose (in all fruits); galactose (in milk); sucrose (made into table sugar); lactose (in milk); and maltose (malt sugar).

Trans-fatty acids: Produced during the manufacture of margarines, these fats behave like saturated fat both in the product (increasing its firmness) and in our bodies (increasing the risk of heart attack). Foods high in trans fats include fried fast foods, some margarines, crackers, cookies and snack cakes.

Triglycerides: The chemical name for fats stored and circulated throughout our bodies.

Vitamin C: An antioxidant vitamin that helps to keep your immune system, capillaries and gums healthy. It is found in such foods as strawberries, oranges, grapefruit, broccoli and green peppers.

Vitamin E: This antioxidant vitamin plays a role in heart health; good food sources include vegetable oils, nuts and seeds.

IF YOU'D LIKE to know the glycemic index of more foods, write to the food manufacturer and encourage them to contact:

SYDNEY UNIVERSITY GLYCEMIC INDEX RESEARCH SERVICE (SUGIRS)

Dr. Jennie Brand Miller
Department of Biochemistry
University of Sydney
NSW 2006 Australia
Fax: (61) (2) 9351-6022
E-mail: j.brandmiller@staff.usyd.edu.au
Website: www.biochem.usyd.edu.au/~jennie/GI/glycemic_index.html

REGISTERED DIETITIANS

Registered Dietitians (RDs) are nutrition experts who provide nutritional assessment and guidance and support for people with heart disease. Check for the initials "RD" after the name to identify qualified dietitians who provide the highest standard of care to their clients. Glycemic index is part of their training so all dietitians should be able to help in applying the principles in this guide, but some dietitians do specialize in certain areas. If you want more detailed advice on glycemic index just ask the dietitian whether this is a specialty when you make your appointment.

Dietitians work in hospitals and often run their own private practices, as well. For a list of dietitians in your area, contact the American Dietetic Association (ADA)'s Consumer Nutrition Hotline (1-800-366-1655) or visit ADAs home page at the address below. You can also check the Yellow Pages under "Dietitians."

THE AMERICAN DIETETIC ASSOCIATION

216 West Jackson Boulevard
Chicago, IL 60606
Phone: 1-800-877-1600
Fax: 1-312-899-1979
Website: http://www.eatright.org/

PRIMARY CARE PHYSICIANS

If you have heart disease or think you may have it, keep in close contact with your primary care physician or heart specialist.

WEIGHT LOSS ORGANIZATIONS

To help you lose weight, check the Yellow Pages under "Weight Control Services." Be aware, however, that not all weight loss organizations are reputable. Check with your physician to make sure the group you'd like to join can help you lose weight safely.

HEART HELP

For more information about the prevention and treatment of stroke, heart disease and related conditions, contact:

THE AMERICAN HEART ASSOCIATION

7272 Greenville Avenue
Dallas, TX 75231
Phone: 1-800-AHA-USA1
Website: http://www.americanheart.org

DIABETES ORGANIZATIONS

Extra weight can often make a diabetic condition worse. For more information about living with and controlling your diabetes, contact the following:

THE AMERICAN DIABETES ASSOCIATION

1660 Duke Street
Alexandria, VA 22314
Phone: 1-800-ADA-DISC (1-800-232-3472)
Web site: http://www.diabetes.org/

CANADIAN DIABETES ASSOCIATION NATIONAL OFFICE

15 Toronto St. Ste. #800
Toronto, ON M5C 2E3
Phone: 1-416-363-3373
1-800-BANTING (1-800-226-8464)
Website: http://www.diabetes.ca/

NATURAL OVENS ORDERING INFORMATION

Natural Ovens of Manitowoc
4300 County Trunk CR
P.O. Box 730
Manitowoc WI 54221-073
Telephone: 1-800-772-0730
Fax: 1-920-758-2594
Website: http://www.naturalovens.com/

ACKNOWLEDGMENTS

We would like to thank Linda Rao, M.Ed., for her enormously valuable editorial work on this edition of the book. We would also like to thank Thomas M.S. Wolever, M.D., Ph.D., for material on monounsaturated fatty acids and high protein diets used in Chapter 4. This material originally appeared in *Nutrition Today*, April 1999. Thanks also to the New South Wales (Australia) Department of Sport and Recreation, the Australian Department of Health and the Australian National Heart Foundation for material on walking for exercise used in Chapter 8.

— JENNIE BRAND-MILLER, KAYE FOSTER-POWELL,
and JOHANNA BURANI
March 2001

light oils, 103
linoleic acid. see omega-6 fatty acid
linolenic acid. see omega-3 fatty acid
linseed oil, 102
lipids, 33, 232
low-density (LDL) cholesterol, 43, 232
"low fat" labels, 26
low G. I. food, 232
    eating, 14–16
    grains and cereals, 91
lunch
    best foods for, 116–117
    weekly menus, 81
lycopene, 58, 232

m

macronutrients, 232
main dishes, recipes, 181–205
mammoth meat, 72
margarine, 20, 23
meal satisfaction, 75
meat, 16
    grain-fed, 21
    lean, ways to prepare, 187
    PUFA content in, 37
Mediterranean diet, 232
    adapting to, 54
    components, 52–53
    fat intake, 43
    healthful effects, 41–42
    low fat diet vs., 45
    micronutrients, 43–44
    study on, 42–43
    typical menu, 55
    vs. Western diet, 53
menus. see also weekly menus
    Asian-style diets, 66
    Mediterranean diet, 55
    Paleolithic diet, 76
metabolism, 232
    human evolution and, 68–69
    insulin and, 12
micronutrients, 232
    Mediterranean diet, 43–44
milk, 10
    PUFA content in, 37
minerals, Paleolithic vs. current intake, 71, 73
monounsaturated fats (MUFAs), 18, 20, 25,
    100, 232
    and dietary guidelines, 52
    diets high in, 46–48
    glucose control, 46–48
    in Mediterranean diet, 42
    oils rich in, 102–103
    in recipes, 133
    sources, 104–105

weight control, 48
motivation, regular exercise, 111
muffins, 223–224

n

nitrosamines, 232
nondairy substitutes, 221–222
noodles, recipes, 167–179
nutrients. see also macronutrients; micronutri-
    ents
    and fullness, 75
    Paleolithic diet, 71, 73
nutrition information, in recipes, 134
nuts, 16
    health benefits, 97
    PUFA content in, 39
    ways to include in diet, 97–98

o

oats, 92
obesity, 4–5
oils, 23
    bad, 21
    cold pressed, 103
    different uses for, 25
    good, 20
    light and extra light, 103
    MUFA-rich, 102–103
    PUFA content in, 35–36
olive oil, 102
    storing, 105
omega-3 fatty acid, 20, 29–30, 33, 232
    concerns with, 32
    content in foods, 35–39
    in fish, 34, 98–99
    food sources, 33
    healthful effects, 30, 31
    oils rich in, 102–103
    and omega-6 ratio, 32
    recipe rating scale, 135–136
    in recipes, 133
omega-6 fatty acid, 20, 33
    content in foods, 35–39
    food sources, 33
    and omega-3 ratio, 32

p

Paleolithic diet, 69, 232
    meat in, 72
    and survival, 72–73
    typical menu, 76
pancreas, 12
pantry foods, 128–129
pasta, 44
    glycemic index table, 225
    recipes, 167–179

peanut oil, 102
peas, 10. see also legumes
    split, 96
phytochemicals, 233
phytoestrogens, 233
polyphenols, 233
polyunsaturated fats (PUFAs), 18, 20, 32,
        100, 233
    content in foods, 35–39
    sources, 104
potatoes, 11
    glycemic index table, 226
pregnancy, omega-3 intake in, 31
protein
    daily servings, 83
    diets high in. see high-protein diet
    Paleolithic vs. current intake, 71, 73
    in recipes, 133, 136
    recommended intake, 25
pumpernickel, 15

r

recipes
    dietary philosophy, 133
    nutrition information in, 134
red kidney beans, 96
"reduced fat" label, 26
refrigerated foods, 130
registered dietitians (RDs), 113–114
rice, 11
    G. I. values, 64–65, 91, 93
    glycemic index table, 227
    types, 62–63
rice wine vinegar, 106
rye, 93

s

salad dressings, PUFA content in, 36
salads, 84
    recipes, 139–166
satiation, 75
saturated fats, 18, 100, 233
    foods high in, 101
    sources, 105
sauces, recipes, 139–166
seafood, 98–99
seeds, PUFA content in, 39
selenium, 59, 233
serving size, 83–84
Seven Countries Study (Mediterranean diet),
        42–43
shoes, 109
shopping, for foods, 128–130
side dishes, recipes, 181–205
snack food
    concealed fat content in, 19

recipes, 139–166
soups
    glycemic index table, 228
    recipes, 139–166
sourdough breads, 15
soy, benefits of, 61–62
soybeans, 61–62
spinach, 86
split peas, 96
sports drinks, 228
sports performance, boosting, 115
spreads, PUFA content in, 35–36
sprouted wheat, 15
squalene, 233
starch
    types, 8
    vegetables, 10
Stone Age diet. see Paleolithic diet
stone ground flour, 15
sugar, 8, 233
survival, diet and, 72–73
sweet potato, preparing, 86

t

tomatoes, 86
tortillas, 16
trans-fatty acids, 22–23, 233
triglycerides, 233

v

vegetable oils. see oils
vegetables, 14
    buying, 86
    colorful variety, 88
    cooking tips, 87
    daily servings, 82, 83
    high intake, benefits of, 58
    preparing, 86
    protective factors, 59, 84
    storing, 86
    ways to include in diet, 85
vinegar, 106
vitamin C, 59, 233
vitamin E, 32, 59, 233
vitamins, Paleolithic vs. current intake, 71, 73

w

walking
    after heart attack or surgery, 111
    frequency and intensity, 109
    healthful benefits, 108, 110
    motivation, 111
    shoes for, 109
    starting, 109
    tips on, 110–111
web sites. see Internet addresses

JENNIE BRAND-MILLER, PH.D., Associate Professor of Human Nutrition in the Human Nutrition Unit, Department of Biochemistry, University of Sydney, Australia, is widely recognized as one of the world's leading authorities on the glycemic index. She received her B.Sc. (1975) and Ph.D. (1979) degrees from the Department of Food Science and Technology at the University of New South Wales, Australia. She is the Editor of the Proceedings of the Nutrition Society of Australia and a member of the Scientific Consultative Committee of the Australian Nutrition Foundation. She has written more than 200 research papers, including 60 on the glycemic index of foods. Her most recent book is the best-selling *The Glucose Revolution*, now in its fully revised second edition, published by Marlowe & Co., in 1999. She lives in Sydney, Australia.

KAYE FOSTER-POWELL, B.SC., M.NUTR. & DIET., is an accredited dietitian-nutritionist in both public and private practice in New South Wales, Australia. A graduate of the University of Sydney (B.Sc., 1987; Masters of Nutrition and Dietetics, 1994), she has extensive experience in diabetes management and has researched practical applications of the glycemic index over the last five years. Her most recent book is the best-selling *The Glucose Revolution*, now in its fully revised second edition, published by Marlowe & Co., in 1999. She lives in Sydney, Australia.

JOHANNA BURANI, M.S., R.D., C.D.E., is a registered dietitian and certified diabetes educator with more than eleven years experience in nutritional counseling. The author of seven books and professional manuals, she specializes in designing individual meal plans based on low G.I. food choices. She lives in Mendham, New Jersey.